# Revitalization Through Transactional Analysis Group Treatment

This innovative book describes the original essence particular to the human species and details the steps necessary to help re-establish this essence, in cases when it has deteriorated, in a therapeutic group context of solidarity and closeness.

Disappointment in primary relationships particularly triggers the deterioration of self-offering, an initially expansive and trusting disposition to affectivity and love. People suffer when, like any fragile and delicate living being early in life, they fail to evolve according to the nature of their species. Therapeutic work is therefore described as mainly oriented to reactivate in a group, a new welcoming family, the original natural drives with new permissions, new trials and new joyful experiences. The book contains the methods and techniques routinely used by the author and two case studies, faithfully transcribed and commented on, particularly for the reactivation of the affective drive.

*Revitatlization Through Transactional Analysis Group Treatment* is an insightful addition to the literature for transactional analysts in practice and in training, for professionals interested in the theory and practice of transactional analysis. Piccinino writes in a compelling manner allowing for the content to be accessible to anyone seeking to understand human processes and wellbeing.

**Giorgio Piccinino** is a sociologist, psychologist, consultant for organizations and psychotherapist in individual, couple and group settings. He is a teacher and supervisor at Schools for Counselors and Psychotherapists and since 1983 a member of national and international associations of Transactional Analysis. He has been a speaker at several conferences and has published six books in Italy.

# Innovations in Transactional Analysis: Theory and Practice

Series Editor: William F. Cornell

This book series is founded on the principle of the importance of open discussion, debate, critique, experimentation, and the integration of other models in fostering innovation in all the arenas of transactional analytic theory and practice: psychotherapy, counseling, education, organizational development, health care, and coaching. It will be a home for the work of established authors and new voices.

**Transactional Analysis of Schizophrenia: The Naked Self**
*Zefiro Mellacqua*

**Groups in Transactional Analysis, Object Relations, and Family Systems: Studying Ourselves in Collective Life**
*N. Michel Landaiche, III*

**Contextual Transactional Analysis: The Inseparability of Self and World**
*James M. Sedgwick*

**New Theory and Practice of Transactional Analysis in Organizations: On the Edge**
*S.J. van Poelje and Anne de Graaf*

https://www.routledge.com/Innovations-in-Transactional-Analysis-Theory-and-Practice/book-series/INNTA

# Revitalization Through Transactional Analysis Group Treatment

## Human Nature and Its Deterioration

Giorgio Piccinino

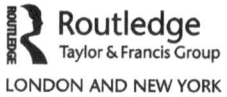

Routledge
Taylor & Francis Group

LONDON AND NEW YORK

Designed cover image: Pitati Bonifacio de' (Bonnifacio Veronese) sec. XVI°.
Private collection Fondazione Federico Zeri, University of Bologna, Italy.

First published 2024
by Routledge
4 Park Square, Milton Park, Abingdon, Oxon OX14 4RN

and by Routledge
605 Third Avenue, New York, NY 10158

*Routledge is an imprint of the Taylor & Francis Group, an informa business*

© 2024 Giorgio Piccinino

*British Library Cataloguing-in-Publication Data*
A catalogue record for this book is available from the British Library

ISBN: 978-1-032-30194-5 (hbk)
ISBN: 978-1-032-30193-8 (pbk)
ISBN: 978-1-003-30383-1 (ebk)

DOI: 10.4324/9781003303831

Typeset in Times New Roman
by SPi Technologies India Pvt Ltd (Straive)

I dedicate this book to Ale, Edo and Guli, my sparkling and joyful family.

# Contents

# Preface

In his latest book, *Human Nature and Its Deterioration: Revitalization Through Transactional Analysis Group Treatment*, Giorgio Piccinino undertakes an extensive reevaluation and vitalization of many of the central concepts in transactional analysis. Here Piccinino writes in a deeply personal and impassioned voice as he articulates a model of TA psychotherapy and counseling that is grounded in a model of personal and interpersonal maturation rather than psychopathology. A sense of the future, of a leaning into the future, of our capacity for becoming more vital human beings pervades this book. There is a moral tone in Piccinino's writing that I, at first as an editor, found disquieting. As I settled into the book and the project Piccinino undertakes here, I realized that this moral perspective is essential to the fabric of the book, grounding his clinical framework is an interweaving of humanistic, existential, and spiritual perspectives.

Giorgio and I worked on his manuscript as the pandemic was slowly coming to an end. In the midst of the profoundly depersonalizing impact of the lockdowns and lives lived virtually on screens, his call – demand really – for a revitalization of human nature could not have been more timely. At a time when we seem increasingly content (resigned) to virtual realities and mediated human contact, there is a particular urgency to the questions and challenges Giorgio puts forth in this book.

Piccinino bookends *Human Nature and Its Deterioration* with deeply personal, transformative accounts of his relationship with his father. His relationship with his father had never been easy, and Piccinino kept a careful distance from his father for much of his life. Through a conversation with his father's brother, he learned for the first time the story of his father's own history and childhood:

> From that moment on I started looking at the world I came from in a different light but, most of all, I started opening my eyes beyond what I could see and understand as a child. From then on, I finally tried to get to know my father. I was 37 …

The invitation to fellow therapists, patients, and all who might read this book to open their eyes beyond those of children is the core of this book. In transactional analysis, the concept of "life scripts" as an enduring and compelling psychological plan for life based in early childhood decisions and beliefs is the ground from which we work. To comprehend the world as perceived and understood by a child is fundamental to psychodynamic forms of treatment. Piccinino does not dispute this, but he underscores the limits of a child's vision and comprehension and the potential for it being over-emphasized, even valorized, during psychotherapy. Instead, he argues that an essential aspect of the therapeutic project is to come to see and embrace our parents as real people with hopes and sufferings of their own – this then being one of the wellsprings of revitalization. The closing chapter of the book is a reflection on his maturing relationship with his father. Piccinino's personal honesty is one of the gifts of this book.

Piccinino's own voice and thinking is intermingled with those of many others – philosophers, cognitive scientists, transactional analysts, researchers, poets, and others who have informed, shaped, and challenged his own thinking, so as to create a rich cascade of voices speaking to both the existential dilemmas of being human and the fundamental creative capacities that make us human. This is a book in which as one reads along, one discovers new authors, repeatedly flipping back to the end to track down the sources of other authors to follow up on. As the editor, I had the rather unusual task of encouraging Giorgio to slow the cascade of voices so that his own voice would be recognized and heard. Through these voices, this book presents a model of psychotherapy that based in the recognition and mobilization of the motivational forces for knowing, self-realization, and belonging.

While it is beyond the purpose of a preface to explore the details of Piccinino's discussion and modifications of TA concepts, I do want to focus briefly on his approach to group treatment, which is central to his work. Eric Berne wrote two seminal books on group theory and group treatment, at the time of their writing being quite radical. Berne had been in training as a psychoanalyst at a time when psychoanalysis was a profoundly dyadic model, one in which there were very clear demarcations between analyst and patient. Berne's work was controversial; he went so far as to experiment with supervision groups attended by both the therapists and their patients, together discussing the successes and difficulties of the therapy. Berne's advocacy for group treatment was a major factor in his being rejected by the psychoanalytic community of the time. Berne's vision was that of patients being fundamentally competent and self-reflective if given the necessary respect and opportunity. This same attitude echoes through Piccinino's detailed accounts of his case examples of his work in groups. Implicit throughout his approach is the message, a persistent and quiet insistence, of the responsibilities of being human enabled through the reflective, revitalizing opportunities of group treatment. A sense of interpersonal and familial care, responsibility, and responsiveness infuses

Piccinino's approach to group treatment. He describes the group as a laboratory for the exploration of one's relational difficulties; as in any laboratory, the
group provides a setting for testing and experimenting with new behaviors and
understandings. Piccinino offers the touching observation that "we are a wonder of dormant opportunities". The group is a rich and experimental field in
which these dormant opportunities may be brought to life.

Piccinino brings the book to a close with his reflections on his father as the
man he came to know and love anew:

> So, when I learned to love my father, I discovered another part of my Parent
> ego state, an assertive, constant, strong, protective parent that exposes him-
> self and fights. And is demanding, very demanding.

Here is the quality of the demand, an invitation and opportunity, to challenge,
extend, and revitalize one's relationship to the intimate others in one's life,
one's parents in particular, and one's own self that unfold through the pages of
this book.

William F. Cornell, M.A., TSTA-ITAA
Editor, Innovations in Transactional
Analysis book series, Routledge

# Acknowledgments

It is really impossible after having written a book like this to make a list of persons to thank. I would have to mention all the persons I met in my life that taught me something, so I'll make a drastic selection.

First of all, I thank the persons who asked me for help and walked with me on their path to growth and transformation, from the first one that I still remember to the last one who phoned me yesterday.

Then the students of the post-graduate schools in psychotherapy and counselling because while teaching one learns a lot.

And then all the friends I more or less drew into my "endeavor".

In particular I thank those who read the drafts of the book and encouraged me to go on. I must say that when I started writing, I didn't know how the book would turn out and therefore it is because of them that this book exists.

Thanks to Delia Duccoli, Dianora Natoli Casalegno, Silvia Pagani, Guido Sicurella, Pierluigi Spatola, and Ivo Setton, who stimulated, corrected and kept focused, advised and applauded me.

Exactly what I needed to keep going.

To Alessandra Cosso my warmest thanks because she did the hardest work: assist me and let me work, bear me and be patient, protect my space and support me and, most of all, remind me of the value of what I was doing. Because in this ambitious and very personal book there is a lot of myself; her courage and her love were indispensable for me to be able to show it.

And love makes miracles!

Aside from the partners of the Center, Anna, Alessandra, Fabio, Gabriela, Giacomo, Pierluigi, and Silvia with whom we integrate and "differentiate" every day, I must also thank in a very special way Alberto Torre, Marco Mazzetti, and Luciano Marchino.

To the last I owe the opportunity of working with "fire", "pain", and "utopia" since he invited me to the seminars organized at the university of Milan Bicocca; my presentations became two chapters of this book but I thank him also for all the conversations that stimulated many original common reflections.

To Alberto Torre, my lifelong supervisor, I owe my love for the persons that come for help, plenty of generosity, and accepting what comes from the world … and many thoughts that I literally copied from him.

To Marco Mazzetti I owe not only sincere friendship but also his constant professional support; his vast and deep expertise in Transactional Analysis has often made up for my ignorance: sometimes a phone call was enough to dispel all my doubts.

I also want to thank all the masters I pillaged in my quotations.

They have been flashes lighting my path that at times seemed to me to be a little risky. But then I thought: if they say so, I can say it too.

With them I saw what the old oriental aphorism says: "A master appears when a student needs him". Suddenly when I was closing the book there appeared Massimo Recalcati with *Le mani della madre*, Rutger Bregman with "De meeste mensen deugen" (*Humankind: A Hopeful History*), William Cornell with *Somatic experience in psichoanalysis and psychotherapy: in the expressive language of the living*, like beacons in the fog that are lighted on the coast, and lastly Irvin D. Yalom with *A matter of death and life*.

The same happened in the past with Raimon Panikkar, Matthew Fox, Telmo Pievani, Massimo Ammaniti, Eugenio Borgna, and Maurilio Orbecchi. They all changed my life.

I am truly grateful to them all.

And last but not least, I express all my gratitude and friendship to Bill Cornell and Marco Mazzetti, who with patience and trust made this English publication possible, and to Daniela Molino who translated this book from Italian in a truly excellent way.

Have I forgotten anyone?

Oh yes, my dad.

Thank you Emilio.

# Chapter 1

# In search of lost time

My father is a strong man, honest, always tidy and clean-shaven, "well groomed" as a bank employee has to be in the 1950s. He is demanding and gruff, often harsh and strict but benign. He is solid and frugal and very ambitious because he always wants to move forward in life and because he cares for me. He wants me to always do the best. When he is outraged by injustice his lips stiffen and he snorts lightly, looking like a bull ready to charge.

He wants to see me safe in life, well accommodated, as he says, meaning married and settled. He doesn't care if I am happy because for him happiness coincides with a solid financial position and that would be already enough.

My father is like this, at least in my memories and my imagination that now, so many years after his death, coincide. But it was not always so.

There were years when it was different for me, years when he was simply my "enemy".

He was the hidden and faraway tyrant to whom my mother told all my deeds so the he could harshly judge them. He was a threatening gaze and impossible to please.

He was the Power that knew all and decided all about me, even what he couldn't possibly know as he was so distant.

But he always knew everything – he used to say that he knew me very well – and this was his way of telling me that he knew even the deepest levels of my foolishness.

At times he was quick-tempered. I was so afraid of him that if I got a bad grade at school my temperature would rise and I ended up in bed even before he came home from work, even before he could punish me.

Once, following some roguery on my part, he smashed the door of my room with a punch.

The hole remained there for months as a warning and a threat of what he could have done if only he decided to turn that dreadful violence on me.

Every once in a while he ran after me if I came back late from the football field near home. He held a broom and when he realized he would not be able to reach me, he threw it at me. Everything turned into a tragedy, and I was often sent to bed without dinner.

DOI: 10.4324/9781003303831-1

When I was a boy he would grab me and turn me upside down in front of his angry eyes holding me by the shoulders so that my head dangled and my disjointed legs banged here and there. While doing this he hurled dark curses on my future saying I was a liar and a loser. Actually I did lie a lot and at school I wasn't certainly among the best. I always thought he was a violent and dangerous man. An enemy, as I said.

How could my mother have married a man like him? On the other hand this is what her whole family thought ... all my maternal aunts. I learned to keep my mouth shut, I never trusted him and kept him at a distance.

I kept away from him but also from my mother. Because she too, despite her joyful and warm attitude, ended up telling him everything. She was kind and affectionate and left to him the double role of public prosecutor and judge.

To do without them was my way to resist, not to submit and to do everything by myself without sharing anything.

In those times parents were almost never on their children's side and my father in particular was for me an omnipotent oppressor, someone you could not turn to and ask for help when needed.

Whatever happened to you was in any case your fault.

I left home as soon as I was able.

At the time I knew nothing of my father's childhood. I only knew he had moved from a village in the mountains of central Italy to a village in the north where he had met my mother.

He was an adolescent when he was sent to live with an old uncle who was a priest and lived in the house annexed to the church. The old priest and the elderly woman attending to his needs spoke only the local dialect while my father spoke his original dialect so at the beginning they barely understood each other. I only knew that he was born in a very poor family with numerous siblings and that all of them, one after the other, had emigrated. He had never mentioned his parents to me.

I was a psychotherapist and lived in a different town from my parents, seldom visiting them when I met one of his brothers who had traveled around the world, enlisted in the navy, and was considered a scoundrel by my father because, unlike him, he was a womanizer, before and after his marriage, and did not love the church. I obviously liked him.

I don't know how we got to it because we did not talk much about the past but once we were alone my uncle spilled all the beans to me in a single sentence:

Our father used to lash us with his belt all the time. He was an ignorant brute and hated to have all these children around. The two things he knew how to do were working and beating us, he wasn't even able to feed all the children he sired. So he got rid of us sending us away when we were still young: your father was sent to the priest, I ran away and found a job on a ship and all our brothers left. I saved myself by joining the navy, I traveled the world and made a career. We were dirt poor and our father was a fuckhead. Your father always respected that pig and defended him and you see what he has become: a servile bigot. He was like that as a child and remained such. A lowly bank employee, a narrow minded little man, compliant and fogy.

I was dumbstruck. I would have never imagined him as submitted and compliant.

I immediately recalled that once I had seen "my threatening enemy" bow to a superior, lowering himself to opening a door for him. I recalled how he was in church. I recalled that he had always been a faithful husband. I recalled that often he skipped his days off and kept working even when our mother took us children to the seaside. I recalled that he always came home from work dead tired and how he had managed with great sacrifice to buy a flat where his children could have a room each, quite rare at the time for families of our social class. I also recalled that he had never actually hit me, neither with the broom nor with his hands.

I looked angrily at my uncle and did not respond but thought that it must have been awful to have a father who cheated on your mother.

From that moment on I started looking at the world I came from in a different light, but most of all, I started opening my eyes beyond what I could see and understand as a child.

From then on I finally tried to get to know my father.

I was 37 and I was truly ashamed for how I had judged him.

I had often despised him but he really did not deserve it.

# Chapter 2

# The fundamental law of nature-physis is the relation

What I understood in many years of experience with the persons that came to me, but also from countless stories I collected in my life, is that in the past few years we stressed the role of fathers and mothers in our society, forgetting that for our happiness and for the full realization of our humanity the role that we played and play toward them as children is just as important.

I could mention many scholars that have recently tackled this subject. from Recalcati (2011, 2013) to Cacciari (2015), Baumann (2005), and Zoja (2009), just to mention a few.

So the question is: when we become adults what do we do with our having been children for our parents?

What do children do with what they learn in relating to their parents?

By developing their Adult Ego State all these Adapted Children, both Natural and Rebellious (to call them with the terms of Transactional Analysis), all these little neurotics, all these great accusers of their parents' atrocities, what can they do to grow up and stop complaining?

How will they treat their parents?

When we are children, we obviously are in their hands and in their arms, but when we are adults do we still go on crying and complaining or will we be able to make a gesture that in nature would be so obvious and very human, like hugging them, in the end, literally, and do something different from what they might have badly taught us?

Will we repeat with them what we have suffered? Will we make them pay for it?

This book wants to help us change this story, look at the past with a compassionate gaze in order for us to make peace with our origins. But it might also have a more ambitious goal: it wants to try to teach us to love our coming in the world, our "generation", to welcome it as a happy event, however it may have been originated.

Love for life and the joy of being alive, even if they have not been our starting point, can become a finishing line.

But then how many sleepless nights are we willing to spend as sons and daughters not just to even out, because that is impossible, but at least to show gratitude for the nights lost by our parents? How much actual and practical

DOI: 10.4324/9781003303831-2

work in terms of caring, supporting, feeding, stimulating, accepting, comforting, protecting, taking to an emergency room and so on, are we willing to do to thank them for having done all this for us (even if badly) and most of all for having brought us into the world? After all, it is thanks to them that we are alive and if we love life … it is thanks to them that we grew up and became what we are.

If we condemn them to oblivion, to indifference, to mere tolerance (sentences and punishments among the worst for a human being; imagine for a parent when they are pronounced by their children), it would mean that we totally despise the life they offered and prepared for us. It would mean that we arrived to the terrible conclusion that they could have spared us the life they gave us. But then we could have taken it as soon as possible, a nice suicide would be a perfect punishment for our parents, as evidence of the evil they produced by bringing us into the world.

Children are not children of one's own parents; they are children of the human species that in that specific year and day, in that specific place, borrowed two bodies and made them join to produce a new life. It is not the parents that give life to their children, obviously more or less accidentally they do, but it is the human species that engages them in mutual attraction and in a sexual imperative in order to survive, propagate, and evolve.

Those children need someone to make them come to life.

So we will look at our parents (they are themselves often unaware of being the tool of something bigger than their will) as the vehicle used by nature to evolve.

The grandiose cosmic nature (or God himself) cannot but look with little interest at who mates with whom and who is born from whom. In the end adults can only decide to avoid to become parents, and with cumbersome maneuvers, but most of their bodies is designed and built for maternity and paternity, much more than for playing tennis or masturbating in front of a video or for singing, praying or painting.

As children we do not choose to be born in a specific family; we get what we get.

It's a game of genes and chance mating, of right temperatures and lucky coincidences; we are born in more or less decorated and welcoming cribs, but we will never know in advance if it was luck for us to enter the richest and most prestigious ones.

There's only one thing that we can do, and this is the deep reason of this book: we can ask whether it's OK for us how we were born and grew and decide then what to do of ourselves.

A patient nearing the end of treatment once told me: "I no longer want to depend on the me I used to be!" Until a short time before seeing me he was only chance and necessity, but then he finally decided to take control of himself and give a direction and a meaning to his existence.

We must not forget that *procreate* means to create for; the aim is always the same for all living beings: to survive as individuals, as communities, as species and to evolve are inevitable necessities.

So writes Fritjof Capra (1996):

Rather than seeing evolution as the result of random mutations and natural selection, we are beginning to recognize the creative unfolding of life in forms of ever-increasing diversity and complexity as an inherent characteristic of all living systems.

(p. 222)

In the same direction go also more recent studies in quantum physics performed by the late Emilio Del Giudice (2007), who dedicated most of his work to proving the condition of resonance in which the Universe is immersed as a single body, inside which are immersed the relation between man and nature and the relations among men. All this scientifically implies a natural ethics and a natural politics that is not individualistic but communal because this is written in the laws of the Universe.

No man can save himself alone neither against nor without other men, neither against nor without the rest of the animate and inanimate world. This vision does not include that insuperable separation between inorganic and living that is the last poisoned fruit of economic liberalism and of a certain type of positivism.

In the technocratic ideology that sustains our often careless progress what is described as the power of man over nature is in fact the power exercised by few men on many men through the undue appropriation of nature.

The universe is expanding, and we are too, but we too are an expression of this law of nature; we are expanding, we are trying to survive, we are taking care of ourselves, we are evolving.

Procreation, the creative unfolding of life, beginning, sympathetic wisdom, archeology of good, resonance, expansion, evolution are some of the new words that have been emerging in the past few years, and we should keep them into account when we discuss what is a human being.

We are born in an affective bubble that is and will be all our life long that archeology of good, wellbeing and happiness that we will always strive to find. It is our extraordinary evolutionary history that provides us with the tools required to recover that original joy and then go on evolving in order to "no longer depend on the us that we were." When we become adults (we hope also as a species because we still have a long road ahead!) we have to choose to maintain the good because we know very well that it is this going against this expansive and cooperative natural ethics that becomes (along with the deterioration of matter, obviously) one of the roots of evil and of human suffering. I think that we should learn to be ecologists also of ourselves, not only as fathers and parents, but also as children and adults because this good is also health and, luckily, as we will see, also happiness.

## Bibliography

Baumann Z. (2005) *Liquid life*. Cambridge, Polity Press.

Cacciari M. (2015) *Re Lear. Padri, figli, eredi* (*King Lear. Fathers, sons, heirs*). Caserta, Saletta dell'Uva.

Capra F. (1996) *The Web of Life*. New York, Doubleday.

Del Giudice E. (2007) Old and New Views on the Structure of Matter and the Special Case of Living Matter. *Journal of Physics Conference Series*, 67: 012006.

Recalcati M. (2011) *Cosa resta del padre? La paternità nell'epoca iper-moderna* (*What's Left of Father? Fatherhood in the hyper-modern age*). Milano, Raffaello Cortina.

Recalcati M. (2013) *Il complesso di Telemaco. Geniori e figli dopo il tramonto del padre* (*The Telemachus Complex. Parents and Children After the Sunset of the Father*). Milano, Feltrinelli.

ZoJa L. (2009) *La morte del prossimo* (*The Death of the Neighbor*). Torino, Einaudi.

# Chapter 3

# Universal drives, the archeology of good

The Human Nature is the outcome of a million years' long run, during which selection yielded an especially resistant but harmless baby, hyperspecialized but fragile, very adaptable and at the same time more and more delicate, potentially full of resources to develop but premature at birth.

We are fragile (I don't like to say weak) and very, very complex.

This living being is extraordinarily equipped with a huge brain, its only weapon for survival, we can say, so large and powerful that it needs years to develop physically and to teach itself how to function: a miracle!

A miracle of balance, always oscillating between automatic actions, unconscious experiences, contradictory propensities, new experiences and choices that we would like to be rational.

Dunbar (2011) calculated, in comparison with animals, the hypothetical gestation time for a human being as related to average life span and to the final formation of the body: we should see the light after 21 months, more or less when we turn one year old (21 – 9 = 12 months). According to evolutionists (Cavalli Sforza, Menozzi and Piazza, 1994) the reason for this (very dangerous) anticipation is due to our adoption of the upright position that induced a relevant narrowing of the pelvis on one side and the progressive and huge growth of the brain on the other.

Two evolutionary adaptations would make the passage of the fetus though the vagina impossible after 21 months, despite the corrective changes consisting in the elasticity of the mother's pelvis and of the baby's cranium.

The incredible width of our rational potential, developed mainly in the prefrontal cortex, started in *Homo sapiens sapiens* over 200,000 years ago (Harari, 2014, 2016), forcing on us premature births. This deprives us of the safety of a physiological growth completed by *Nature*, and puts our immature bodies in the hands of the maternal and family *Culture* to complete our growth.

Many of our difficulties and sufferings derive precisely from all the learning and adapting we have to go through while our brain cells are still totally unprotected from the messages from the environment and are certainly unable to rationally orient our actions (Dehaene et al. 2005) [eds.] *From Monkey Brain to Human Brain*. Cambridge, MA: MIT Press).

DOI: 10.4324/9781003303831-3

We are no longer only in the hands of our nature; we are in the hands of our parents when we are still dangerously incomplete, and they are often unprepared. From a certain point of view, it is as if half of a Ferrari had been designed and built by extremely expert engineers and then was left in the hands of amateurs who have to complete it. Can we imagine what happens to our perception of the world and of ourselves, to our trust, to our stability, to our propensity to love in those first months of care?

At a certain point *Homo sapiens* became *Sapiens sapiens*, but because of this also became full of doubts and uncertainties, unaware of his fragility and mortality, of his ignorance and probably most of all of how his destiny was mostly in the hands of chance (Tomasello, 1999, 2008).

But why did we do this? Evolutionists do not have a definite answer yet but probably (Cavalli and Pievani, 2011, Harari, 2014) we did it to survive and for a series of factors: a persistent lack of food, a too fast population increase, or the arrival of invasive and dangerous predators; maybe all these factors combined forced us to seek a future out of Africa (and in many different ways).

All in all this is still happening in many regions of the world; we try to survive with any means and anywhere.

But let's move one step at a time.

Three different species of anthropomorphic great apes of the genus *Homo*, the *ergaster* (1.5 million years ago), *heidelbergensis* (200,000 years ago) and *sapiens* (125,000 and then 85,000 years ago) came out of Africa at intervals of hundreds of years, not an especially curious and active Lucy as once was thought, but many generations in subsequent waves moved North, East, West, leaving from scattered areas of Africa. Many of these groups did not survive (Calzolaio and Pievani, 2016).

They came down from trees four-handed and after a few thousand years became bipeds so that their hands were free and they could look in the distance and protect themselves from aggressors with objects more powerful than their hands.

But how did they defend themselves? On trees the automatic (instinctive) system for defending themselves from predators was closing their eyes, freezing, camouflaged in foliage, lifting their hands to protect their faces. Today this is still the more or less immediate response of a newborn to danger.

Here too I cannot imagine the shock of protecting oneself in this way in the open, in the savanna, in front of hungry carnivores. How many must have died before someone brilliant "invented" a new mental function, something that could go against a million-year-old automatic response and substitute it with another behavior.

To flee, to run and then to strike alliances and form groups, then build arms, and traps, and fences and then anticipate and assault, then build and cultivate. And then teach others to do all this.

It took us millions of years to learn how to survive anywhere without predefined instincts and to learn to think rationally according to situations.

Old automatic responses do not disappear but are only used less frequently, leaving room to other ones that seem more adequate for survival (Cavalli Sforza, Menozzi and Piazza, 1994).

These considerations might not seem so relevant but they are crucial according to those who study human behavior: the old automatic actions do not disappear, neither the individual nor the species-specific ones.

This is also one of the reasons why the brain developed so much it had to grow in spirals and circumvolutions and troughs and recesses; it had to grow upon itself in order not to explode and become impossible to keep on top of the neck. So a *mind* had to develop that is capable of thinking itself, of reflecting on its behaviors and on its functioning, capable of exchanging information fast within itself, a mind "scattered" in interconnected areas of the brain ready to send signals of danger and fear and rage and pain and wellbeing in order to inform its own operating and decision centers. For generations we have learned and stored complex sequences of sensations, emotions, thoughts, behavioral styles to respond to the various needs coming from the outside and at the same time realize our drives and vital needs.

One of the most important cognitivist experimental scientists, Stanislas Dehaene (2014) writes:

> The richness of information processing that an evolved network of sixteen billion cortical neurons provides lies beyond our current imagination. Our neuronal states ceaselessly fluctuate in a partially autonomous manner, creating an inner world of personal thoughts. Even when confronted with identical sensory inputs, they react differently depending on our mood, goals, and memories. Our conscious neuronal codes also vary from brain to brain. Although we all share the same overall inventory of neurons coding for color, shape, or movement, their detailed organization results from a long developmental process that sculpts each of our brains differently, ceaselessly selecting and eliminating synapses to create our unique personalities.
>
> (p. 265)

Is it surprising that such a complexity can easily get stuck, deteriorated, reduced and most of all confused? Is it surprising that we develop neuroses, psychoses, and psychopathologies and therefore we are beset by bloody tyrants, serial killers, lecherous and corrupt politicians and in turn by psychiatrists, psychotherapists, priests, lawyers and policemen and magistrates?

As we will see later on, we obviously select a few of these billions of mental pathways, then we pave and fence them in order to use them more frequently and fast, to simplify and economize once and for all our mental reference frame and our choices (what we call Script in TA).

This is a way to defend ourselves from this unbearable complexity with the relevant problem of creating new limiting rigidities, behaviors that are hard to change. Such a vast sea of possibilities becomes at times so scary that leads many disoriented minds to drastically reduce their and their children's free will options to a level of mere survival.

This is what often happens to small and uncertain minds who then end up following a leader or a tyrant delegating to them the choices that they are unable to make.

We know a selection of possible behaviors is inevitable as is the creation of relevant automatic actions, but this will create a new problem for human beings: what will be the quantity, quality, precocity and "definitiveness" of the reduction of possibilities made in infancy?

I believe it is important to explore the use we make of this complexity, because the drastic reduction of the instinctual constraints to mere propensities helps us to be free to act in modes that we choose according to the problems we encounter, to invent machines that are more and more complex for making our life more comfortable, to ward off death, to face fear, to recover if we are ill, to avoid suffering.

But it should help us also to be happy and give a meaning to our existence.

The Existential psychotherapeutic school describes the main goals of human beings as follows (Yalom, 2002).

- To accept the inevitability of death, ours and that of our loved ones
- To be free to determine our life through our personal choices
- To manage loneliness in the world
- To give a meaning and a sense to our existence

So the mind should serve our survival, and for this reason it organized its vital energy in information systems and behavioral patterns in different interconnected areas genetically transmitted and consolidated after millions of years of evolution. Newborn babies already have a predisposition to become a human being; they are physiologically and psychologically premature but with orientations to action ready to be triggered, if they are welcomed and supported, in order to play their part in the world.

In the same sense Maurilio Orbecchi, in his enlightening preface to Pierre Janet's new Italian publication *La psicoanalisi* (2014), reminds us that:

Janet's tendencies to action … are so important and up to date that they are being recovered by various schools of psychology and psychoanalysis. One of the distinguished psychologists that theorized ex novo the tendencies to action … was again John Bowlby who wrote about "behavioral systems

and Internal Operating Models. Later cognitive psychologists called them Modules and developmental psychologists called them "psychological mechanisms." Some groups in current psychoanalysis revisited this part of Janet's and Jackson's work and redefined the tendencies to action with the term "motivational systems" (p. 45).

Human beings are born vital and energetic, endowed with an original tendency to action, the mentioned motivational systems, to keep themselves alive and reproduce.

Exploring these issues in depth, I found Raimon Panikkar's (2005) approach very interesting. He was a theologian capable of moving with total freedom among the dogmas of the most important religions, among ancient and modern cultures in various continents, among different languages and literatures. He was able to synthetize an overarching intercultural theory of the values common to populations. He called them the four centers of wisdom, in perfect coincidence with the archetypes of Earth, Wind, Water, and Fire with some drive areas that can be called Survival, Love, Knowledge, and Self-Realization.

I started out calling these features "existential orientations" (Piccinino, 2000, 2006) while the philosopher and psychoanalyst Umberto Galimberti called them "general urges to an indeterminate aim", the philosopher and evolutionist Telmo Pievani (2014) called them "propensities", the doctor, anthropologist and psychotherapist Maurilio Orbecchi, "natural precursors" (2015) and the psychotherapist Joseph Lichtenberg (1989) "motivational systems".

However, it seems that except for some minor adjustments we barely moved from the theory of needs presented by Maslow in the 1950s that highlighted the deep motivations of human beings (Maslow, 1954) or even earlier (1913) the "tendencies to action" of the great psychoanalyst Janet, later marginalized.

If we wanted to be precise we should say that human beings are born with orientations that are neither needs nor shortfalls but evolutionarily determined activities that are indispensable to survival. A set of abilities that need to be developed and made realizable that are however propensities well identifiable in all infants that are expressed autonomously by each baby according to rhythms that follow the growth from embryo to adult being.

Need is instead aimed at finding stimuli, recognitions, and structures (Berne, 2000), which means confirmations, support, containments, limitations, and organization to learn how to rationally manage drives. So, drives are different from needs as in own way, Freud (1915) himself first hypothesized (Imbasciati, 2005).

This distinction may sound like sophistry but it will prove quite relevant if we apply it to what is considered most important in this book: to analyze and take care of the affective drive that is first and foremost a primary autonomous activity of each and all human beings, exactly like developmental energy and survival.

Another distinction that I mentioned above needs to be stressed before proceeding and concerns the difference between Instincts and Drives. In the course of millennia, animals either became extinct or adapted and changed while "adaptively winning" behaviors consolidated into instincts as did their bodies. (https://desistenza.wordpress.com/2017/02/08/istinto-e-pulsione/)

Evolutionists explain that human beings in their constant peregrinations had to renounce this rigid behavioral consolidation and kept only a few basic features that had to find ample scope for expression in different behaviors according to the different environments they inhabited. For us culture took up an extraordinary role so that we learned how to apply these (former) instincts that had become generic propensities, moldable according to necessity, becoming what we now call tendencies to action (Stenhouse, 1974).

It should be noted, however, that already in the 1800s Darwin wrote about these differences with animals explaining that they were differences in degree rather than in quality: more evolved animals too are sad or angry if they are mistreated or "forced against their nature", they too learn and can choose between various behavioral options. We could say that they are only a little behind us in evolutionary terms, but affectivity and intelligence are certainly not an exclusive feature of humankind.

We could also say that these tendencies to action are fragile instincts. Just as an example, think of how in some schools we mortify the drive to learn or to creativity.

So, at birth we are ready to speak as we are ready to love and learn but only if these propensities are welcomed, supported and progressively turned into action through the examples and teachings of caregivers.

In order to survive, human beings first of all discovered group living, as did many other animals obviously, but apart from the fact that we can choose to do it or not, with the great difference that the link that is no longer forced must be supported by affectivity, by loving. And therefore we must say that the drive is not to living in a group but primarily that to affective attachment to another (Bowlby, 1979).

Many scholars and researchers call this co-belonging in order to stress the importance of the co-specific link (Coon, 1946, Eibl-Eibessfeldt, 1989, Baumeister and Leary, 1995).

We are born in love and affectively oriented to others, we feel joy in attachment with our fellow humans, we are born generous and altruist (Tomasello, 2014) and naturally good (De Waal, 2001) or, as Mancuso (2013) would put it, oriented to good with an extraordinary ability to share and understand the emotions and actions of others.

As the discovery of mirror neurons is showing, we empathically take part in the lives of others with "bio-social" behaviors that precede any linguistic communication (Rizzolatti and Sinigaglia, 2006).

We are predisposed to love and phylogenetically this precedes our becoming individuals: we are together before being alone. But it is important to stress that this does not exclude that if we feel we are in danger we are capable of responding in order to survive, attacking and killing even our fellow humans. When our survival drive clashes with the belonging drive, it is usually the former to prevail.

Still we are born in symbiosis with our mother's body, a body that is available to us, warm and reassuring, and provides all we need to be born. The fetus lives with that body in a substantial state of general wellbeing until the moment of separation, physical and psychological, and from that initial state of wellbeing the fetus "sees" the mother for the first time. And smiles to her not in response to her smile (even blind babies do that, Fraiberg, 1999), but as a proposition of affective link, it is the affective drive that is always directed to the first fellow human that is recognized as such. We love co-specific others before we are born, just like a cub monkey is afraid of and avoids snakes and hairy spiders even before seeing them.

There exists an unknown world that belongs to us even before we are born.

From their very first utterance, babies offer themselves to contact; they are not passive. They offer affection, approaching and exploration motions. They start with that woman a dance made of mutual recognitions and mirrorings that should be confirmed and supported (Ammaniti and Gallese, 2014). The newborns offer their affection as an instinctive motion of trusting and unconditioned belonging because this kind of link has always been for humankind a crucial factor for successful survival and a very powerful comforting system against anxiety, fear and pain both in the baby-caregiver link and in the community.

This offer of a peaceful and affective relation is embedded in our deepest nature.

Altruism (De Waal, 1996, Tomasello, 2009, Pievani, 2014, the sense of justice (De Waal, 1991), the concept of common good, sociability and, for larger groups, the need to protect communal life with rules and regulations (Nowak and Highfield, 2011) have always been features of humankind even though less constraining (unfortunately) than for many other animals.

Along with the belonging drive another extraordinary propensity for our evolution started consolidating somewhere in our DNA the drive to be oneself, individuation, differentiation, the foundation of a peculiar identity for many aspects different from that of all the others. After a few weeks of life, the newborn discovers the Other, discovers themselves as separate from the body that contained and nurtured them and smiles happily.

Think of what developmental leap humankind must have made when someone realized that they could act differently from their group; think of what changes this condition can have caused. The consequences are found mainly in the area of creativity; think also of how many lives have been saved in dangerous situations by the adoption of new more appropriate behaviors in front of new threats.

But from this same propensity derives also the tendency to act as one wishes, to realize oneself as an individual and to express oneself (art therefore) and the awareness of our mortal condition and the search for answers to questions that only we humans are aware of (spirituality).

Why do we live? To what end? What is there after death? Questions that children start to ask quite early.

A last drive, just as necessary for a species that is not so thick-skinned and rather poor in defenses, is the propensity to learn: we are born curious, we want to learn, we try to grow and become capable to make our mind work.

The potential of our brain, as we know, is boundless and countless as are the pieces of useful information that make it work; this is why the duration of the phase of training that humans undergo before becoming adults has no equal in nature. For this reason we live with our family for so many years. We employ about a quarter of our life to become independent and capable of looking after ourselves when a cat or a dog employs a fifteenth of it and a butterfly, a frog, or an insect a tiny percentage: they are born and they are basically already adults; they don't need to learn much after birth: what they need is already included in their very specialized instinctual makeup.

Think of the power of the whys our children ask, think of their vivacity and curiosity, think of their tirelessness in asking for explanations. Think of how every newborn repeats ontogenetically the evolution of all humankind, think of how every stage of our growth is foreseen with very small differences in all human cultures and in all races (Eibl-Eibessfeldt, 1989), think of how in any part of the world the *esprit vitale* is deployed in the very same way with similar gestures and an emotional support mechanism that is initially virtually perfect.

Our nature is therefore energetic, reproductive, defensive/aggressive (the SUR-VIVAL drive); altruistic, trusting, cooperative, loving (the BELONGING drive); curious, exploring, longing for knowledge, intelligent (the EVOLUTION drive); differentiated, individual, self-centered, spiritual (the SELF-REALIZATION drive).

Research in the fields of neuroscience and experimental psychology is heading in this same direction. Panksepp and Biven (2012) for example identified six affective instinctive basic systems (endophenotypes) that are found in all human beings. We feel these systems without reflection and we build our conscious mental life on them: exploration/search, lust, need for caring, caring and affection, pain, fear/anger in front of obstacles to life and social play. I think this description mixes propensities and emotions, behaviors and internal sensations, but I mention it because I want to stress that the drive constants can be named and grouped in different ways, but it is very evident that inside us there are different psychobiological systems that are interconnected and can be isolated from the functioning of the neocortex and of the rational control systems.

Always in this area it is worth mentioning also the self-determination theory by Deci and Ryan (1985, 2000), cognitive behavioral scientists at the University of Rochester in the USA who studied the intrinsic motivations of human beings and defined them as self-determined active organisms oriented to realizing in a consistent and balanced way three innate needs: competence (knowledge/evaluation), autonomy (self-realization) and relation (belonging).

As we can see we are perfectly in line with the drives mentioned above. It is important to stress that for these authors too the behaviors oriented to meeting these needs do not necessarily require reinforcement or reward; they are in fact acted in themselves provided one sees the possibility of succeeding.

I think therefore that a psychotherapist should keep in mind, more than has been done so far, our "first" nature. We must consider our nature as marvelous and our propensities as a treasure to be protected because it will more and more be our responsibility to preserve this "great beauty" that struggles in the uncertain and often deteriorated hands of a mother, a father, a teacher, in short a culture.

These are our vital propensities and their realization is the aim of our existence and in the end the essence of our humanity.

I believe that newborn babies today should be considered the peak of our developmental history, their nature should be considered sacred and it should be a taboo to intervene for changing and limiting it because it is so since the great leap forward.

When we hold them in our arms, we should always be aware of their fragility, of their precocity, of their dependence on our responses to grow well and remain healthy.

A relevant part of my work as psychotherapist is, as we will see in detail below, an activity aimed at recovering the natural propensities that have not been welcomed in early life or that have progressively deteriorated. In the past few years, not only in the West, the great rush to a huge and not well-regulated growth that privileged a few and damaged multitudes has become a more and more nervous and breathless whirlwind that generates anxiety and depersonalizes at staggering psychological costs. This worldwide competition among peoples and individuals increasingly neglects one of the deepest *essences* of human beings: happy affectivity and joy of living.

## Bibliography

Ammaniti M., Gallese V. (2014) *The Birth of Intersubjectivity. Psychodynamic, Neurobiology, and Self*. New York, W. W. Norton & Co.

Baumeister R.F., Leary, M. R. (1995) The need to belong: Desire for interpersonal attachments as a fundamental human motivation. In *Psychological Bulletin*, 117.

Bowlby J. (1979) *The Making and Breaking of Affectional Bonds*. London, Routledge.

Calzolaio V., Pievani T. (2016) *Libertà di migrare: Perché ci spostiamo sempre ed è bene così* (*Freedom to migrate: Why we're always moving and it's okay to do so*). Torino, Einaudi.

Cavalli Sforza L., Menozzi P., Piazza A. (1994) *The History of Geography of Human Genes*. Princeton, NJ, Princeton University Press.

Cavalli Sforza L., Pievani T. (2011) *Homo sapiens. La grande storia della diversità umana* (*Homo Sapiens. The Grand Story of Human Diversity*). Torino, Codice.

Coon C. (1946) The universality of natural groupings in human societies. In *The Journal of Educational Sociology*, 20(3).

De Waal F. (1991) The chimpanzee's sense of social regularity and its relation to the human sense of justice. In *American Behavorial Scientist*, 34(3): 335–349.

De Waal F. (1996) *Good Natured: The Origins of Right and Wrong in Humans and Other Animals*. Cambridge US, Harvard University Press.

Deci E. L., Ryan R. M. (1985) *Intrinsic Motivation and Self-Determination in Human Behavior*. New York, Plenum Press.

Deci E. L., Ryan R. M. (2000) The "what" and "why" of goal pursuits: Human needs and the self-determination of behavior. In *Psychological Inquiry*, 11: 227–268.

Dehaene S. (2014) *Consciousness and the brain: Deciphering How the Brain codes Our Thoughts*. New York, Viking Press.

Dehaene, S. Duhamel, J. R., Hauser, M., Rizzolatti, G. (2005) *From Monkey Brain to Human Brain*. Cambridge, MA. MIT Press.

Dunbar R. (2011) *How many friends does one person need?* London, Faber & Faber.

Eibl-Eibesfeldt I. (1989) *Human Ethology*. New York, Routledge.

Fraiberg Selma H. (1999) *Il sostegno allo sviluppo (Development support)*. Milano, Raffaello Cortina.

Harari Y. N. (2014) *Sapiens: A Brief History of Humankind*. London, Harvill Secker.

Harari Y. N. (2016) *Homo Deus: A Brief History of Tomorrow*. London, Harvill Secker.

Imbasciati A. (2005) *La sessualità e la teoria energetico pulsionale: Freud e le conclusioni sbagliate di un percorso geniale, (Sexuality and Drive Energy Theory: Freud and the Mistaken Conclusions of a Brilliant Path)*. Milano, Franco Angeli.

Janet P., Orbecchi M. (2014) *La psicoanalisi (Psychoanalysis)*. Torino, Bollati Boringhieri.

Lichtenberg, Joseph D. (1989) *Psychoanalysis and Motivation*. New York, Routledge.

Mancuso V. (2013) *Il principio passione. (The Passion Principle)*. Milano, Garzanti.

Maslow A. (1954) *Motivation and Personality*. London, Harper & Row.

Nowak M., Highfield R. (2011) *SuperCooperators: Altruism, Evolution, and Why We Need Each Other to Succeed*. New York, Free Press.

Orbecchi M. (2015) *Biologia dell'anima. Teoria dell'evoluzione e psicoterapia. (Biology of the Soul. Evolutionary Theory and Psychotherapy)*. Torino, Bollati Boringhieri.

Panikkar R. (2005) *La dimora della saggezza (The Abode of Wisdom)*. Milano, Mondadori.

Panksepp J., Biven L. (2012) *The Archeology of Mind. New York. Neuroevolutionary Origins of Human Emotions*. New York, W. W. Norton & Company.

Piccinino G. (2000) *La forza del destino. (The Power of Destiny)*. Napoli, Dinosauro.

Piccinino G. (2006) *Il piacere di lavorare. (The Pleasure of Working)*. Trento, Erickson.

Pievani T. (2014) *Evoluti e abbandonati. (Evolved and Abandoned)*. Torino, Einaudi.

Rizzolatti G., Sinigaglia C. (2006) *So quel che fai. Il cervello che agisce e i neuroni specchio (I Know What You Do. The Acting Brain and Mirror Neurons)*. Milano, Raffaello Cortina.

Stenhouse D. (1974) *The Evolution of Intelligence*. New York, Barnes & Noble Books.

Stern D. (1995) *Motherhood Constellation: A Unified View of Parent-Infant Psychotherapy*. New York. Routledge.

Tomasello M. (1999) *The Cultural Origins of Human Cognition.* Harvard University Press. Cambridge, USA.

Tomasello M. (2008) *Origins of Human Communication*, Cambridge, MA, MIT Press.

Tomasello M. (2009) *Why We Cooperate*, Cambridge, MA, MIT Press.

Tomasello M. (2014) *A Natural History of Human Thinking.* Cambridge, MA, Harvard University Press.

Yalom I. (2002) *The gift of therapy: an open letter to a new generation of therapists and their patients.* New York, Harper Collins.

# Chapter 4

# How human nature deteriorates

At the beginning of life there is almost always a pleasant sense of protection, a healthy symbiosis where all the things a baby needs for surviving are made available by the more or less unvoluntary functioning of a mother.

I ought to say from the start that this functioning works better and is mutually satisfying if the mother-baby couple is protected and surrounded by the attention first of all of her partner and of her community. The role of the partner and of society is crucial for an experience of love and calm in the present and in the future, to facilitate the mother in donating herself to the fetus and later to the newborn.

The miracle of budding life requires peace, stability, unconditional acceptance, an exclusive link, at least in the first period and preferably for the whole first year of life not because the baby needs a total and continuous presence but to guarantee constant care and timeliness in catching the baby's verbal and non-verbal signs of need, pain and, let's not forget it, insecurity.

In TA we talk of Unconditional Love to name that set of messages babies should receive to continue to feel welcome and accepted and at the same time to grow stronger in a loving and benevolent world. This is what we call structuring not only of a safe base but also of a perception of the Other from oneself as loving and benevolent.

Thus: not only I am OK, but you too are OK.

It is easy to think that the whole community should be part of this, not only the mother.

Two are the persons physically and mentally involved in birth and therefore two, mother and baby obviously, are the persons that need to be supported and protected and kept untroubled and not for six months, one or two years ...!

Read how Jared Diamond describes the world where the highly developed Guineans (and they are certainly well beyond us) take care of maternity. It makes you wish to leave all here and move there to have children. The serenity, kindness and gentleness of attitudes, the basic calm, inner peace and warmth of all the adults are born there: in a community activated to support maternity as the first essential element for the survival and psycho-physical wellbeing of individuals and of the whole community.

DOI: 10.4324/9781003303831-4

First of all, we must guarantee the fulfillment of the survival drive since certainly newborns will not be able for many years to guarantee it by themselves. However, it must be clear that for us human survival must be seen also from a psychological point of view because our physical wellbeing depends very much on our emotional and affective wellbeing and therefore on the acceptance, love, recognition that will keep supporting the constant progressive emergence of our propensities.

Human drives emerge and urge to action constantly and cyclically during childhood: in a few hours the baby can feel a lack of protection and therefore activate their survival and belonging drives; in other circumstances they feel the urge to explore the world and look everywhere. Time for children is marked by explorative behaviors like in a familiar gym where they look for confirmations and limits and where they learn the abilities required for the autonomous fulfilment of each drive.

For each drive babies will structure specific neuronal circuits, organizational schemes of self-standing behaviors, emotions, and thoughts that will be repeated in time until they become "Ego States", automated and more or less consistent with the essence of human nature. And more or less aware.

For each drive we will feel more or less happiness, will receive more or less rewards and praise. For each of them in the end we will think we are more or less talented so that we will unconsciously orient our life to the fulfillment of one rather than the other. And it will be quite often a ranking already inscribed in the family's Script.

### The most dangerous pain, not being allowed to exist (and being OK)

The messages of love, welcome and acceptance to the baby for what they are ("you are OK as you are") solidify their right to be in the world, implant indelibly an experience of possible happiness in the innermost archaic neural circuits, confirm the joy of being in the world, stabilize the trust that the Other is a friend, a fellow human being, guarantee that their primary needs can be met and that after the inevitable crying there will always be a smile, help, satisfaction, peace. The loving responses, joyful mirrorings, assenting smiles, the festive dance (Stern, 1987, 1995) of stimuli and responses, discoveries and frustrations, trials and errors, confirm to the babies that they are also (and foremost) bearers of happiness, that they are able to give love and joy.

It is this wonderful world that a baby should meet, this is the first right, the right to life, to a healthy and cared for life, basically stable, safe and protected, if not always pleasant but easily brightened.

As I said, it is difficult that a mother does not accompany in this way her pregnancy and later her caring for her newborn baby; in general the risk of inadequacy steps in after the body has played its part. Often a less healthy and less altruistic part prevails in the management of behaviors and can send deeply destructive messages, of rejection or of manic caring, that contradict deeply what the baby has perceived until then.

I want to stress and highlight this passage that will be very important for psychotherapeutic work with adults.

I say it now: a baby is traumatized always by disappointment.

It is this change that "hits" the baby: to move from total caring to indifference, to rejection, makes them suspect that they have done something wrong or that they have disappointed, that they are no longer the baby that their mother wanted, in sum, that they are not right.

The baby will respond to the lack of care by feeling unloved even if this perception is almost never totally true! The earlier and more drastic the mother's change of attitude, the more catastrophic the baby's experience will be. Not to mention the case of possible malnutrition, physical abandonment, violence, that always affect psychophysical and neuronal development when occurring in the first months of life.

These are obviously the most serious and heavy damages that take place when the baby perceives a sense of total inadequacy without a possible explanation.

The words that we can give during treatment to recover this experience of not being welcome are clearly arbitrary. In this phase, in fact, lack of care and absence are perceived in the body and emotionally by the baby through the caregiver's nonverbal messages that are recorded in implicit memory.

Words are not yet recorded because cognitive memory has not yet had time to develop enough to remember and give a name to this early distress. It is therefore not something "repressed", as is often suggested, but of something "unthought known" (Bollas, 1982) because, as Orbecchi (2015) also reminds us: "we know that until the third year of life the memory circuits are not yet developed: early experiences dating back to the first and second year of life, the most important ones, normally cannot be remembered."

Words will come later on and will confirm and give voice and content to those family attitudes that will be probably repeated also later on. These messages are "Injunctions" to not exist and carry with them deep consequences at various psychopathological levels. There is no doubt, however, that frustrating, rejecting, abandoning, aggressive interventions against the survival drive can cause some of the most severe even if not necessarily immediate responses from a psychological point of view.

Each baby responds in their own way, adapting or opposing or retreating. In any case they will find some sort of protective strategy even if paying a high price to save themselves from the anxiety of having been abandoned.

If mother forgets them for hours, they will do without her; if mother is violent, after a while they will surrender; if they are beaten, they will submit; if treated with indifference, they will manage by themselves; if mother is distressed and depressed, they will take care of her; if they are not seen, they will let themselves be seen with provocative or hyperkinetic behaviors; and so on.

In this way they will learn to "survive" literally in their specific way that is no longer healthy.

The general premise will be "I am not OK, but you, mother, are OK", the premise behind all the pathological responses on the depressive side: I am the one who is not right.

The other large part of early pathological responses, on the paranoid side, is the answer: "You are not OK, I am only your sacrificial victim, but you won't get me!" with a rebellious and angry reaction that ends up trying to pass the inadequacy from oneself to the Other, at least superficially. But it is much more probable that the conclusion, or the suspicion, is "I am not OK, but you too aren't doing well, you are not OK" a catastrophic and distressing view where no one is saved.

If a baby does all this to survive, not to fall apart, they will manage with defensive behaviors (offensive behaviors are a defense too) to survive.

In these conditions they will neither be calm nor happy but at least in this determined and aggressive, alarmed and suspicious responsiveness they will remain alive and energetic, seen and recognized with a personal identity. These are "survival" behaviors that will become their main way of facing life, the Script on which to stabilize the perception of the world and the best behaviors to face it: "now I know how to get the attention I need in this situation, now I know who I am".

## The deepest inconsolable pain, not being allowed to love

As I mentioned at the beginning of this book, based on my clinical experience but even more on the countless statements of scholars of different disciplines (for example, Sennet, 2012, Stern, 1995, Bowlby, 1979, 1988, Pievani, 2014, Brooks, 2011, Nowak and Highfield, 2011), I am convinced that peoples capable of cooperating are better at surviving and that the co-belonging drive is based on a primary relational affective impulse. A smile is probably the first sign of communication to the Other, expressing the joy deriving from meeting a fellow human, indispensable for survival. Human communication, let us never forget it, is born first of all as an expression of oneself, an action that signals and expresses a state of pleasure, joy, and recognition or of fear or aggression.

Smiling precedes by millennia any intentional word, is the evidence of an internal state of joy welcoming a fellow human, is an offering of dialogue and of possible and wished for closeness, a gesture of alliance and favor (Borgna, 2013).

A smile is not a reflection of mother's smile (Fraiberg, 1999) but is the affective drive that settles on the first fellow human the baby recognizes and is grateful to and to which they attach in order to survive. This is why it is so difficult to fake a smile; one can bend the mouth but if the smile is not truthful, the eyes do not express authentic joy and remain opaque and cold. With the development of the prefrontal cortex and of reflective and discriminating abilities such gestures become willful and addressed to a finalized communication. But in the meantime through those first relations, we learn to love without realizing it.

The modes we use are all cultural and depend on the shaping in our mind of a model of intersubjectivity, initially just dual and exclusive, that will progressively expand toward all other fellow humans.

In the first years of life, we acquire the abilities indispensable for fulfilling this propensity and we learn:

- Whether being loved is a right or we need to earn it through specific behaviors (the Script Drivers that we will see later: Be Strong, Be Perfect, Be Complying, Strive, Hurry);
- Whether we can confidingly surrender in the arms of the Other and loving will be easy;
- Whether our beauty can be enjoyed by the Other or we need to hide it;
- Whether we can show ourselves without fear;
- Whether we can be intimate and authentic;
- Whether the Other is friend or foe;
- Whether we can sensuously enjoy physical contact, acceptance and mutual hugs;
- Whether we will be able to repeat the modes of parental love that we learned, even only as imitation, such as a dedicated care of others and ourselves;
- Whether we will be able to ask for help or to find consolation and sharing with others;
- Whether we will look at strangers with different degrees of curiosity and attention;
- Whether we will be able to defend ourselves or repel.

All life-long a healthy overcoming of the exclusive and symbiotic dependence from mother will also mean to develop a balance of the propensities to differentiation and self-assertion and will provide an indelible trace for a possible relational happiness. To progressively leave our safe base, to return to it and be welcomed after an exploration, to get to know new attachment and identification figures, to feel free and capable of moving, to be able to establish and leave relationships, to discover new affects, are all situations that will favor emotions of joy and satisfaction and will foster the growth of self-esteem and confirm the right to love, affectivity, thankfulness, and relational joy all life-long.

The abilities required to adults for a satisfying affective and relational life are many: negotiations, empathic communication, kindness, ethics, sense of justice, cooperativeness, generosity, the ability to comfort, to contribute to growth, optimism, and the like. But most of all we will confirm our innate "human warmth", the undefinable contact that allows us to get near someone without invading them and to welcome them without detaining them.

And then respect for the dignity of all human beings.

The constant exercise of this propensity during childhood will give us such a joy that it will be hard for us to give it up. We will always feel a deep longing for those hugs, that sweet and trusting surrender, that getting lost in a fusion that is pleasant and nourishing. Our senses will be enhanced by it, our skin will have a memory of it, and we'll always listen with sweet nostalgia to a song or a lullaby, we will know how to care, touch, kiss, and embrace. We will know how to make love.

Then we will have a definitive confirmation that we belong to humankind in a link that is common to all in the most difficult moments of our living on this earth.

There are quite a number of abilities that we need to learn how to use in order to fulfill the belonging drive, and we might meet just as many difficulties.

We are truly complex and delicate, it seems that a true "miracle" is necessary for everything to work properly in the first years of life without receiving inhibitory messages (injunctions) that tell us not to belong, not to be intimate, not to love, but also not to feel and not to share. Messages that can obviously not be related to a disturbed or cold behavior of our mother; I am thinking for example of some inevitable separations due to illness or very poor material conditions that can lead to a separation of some children from their parents that is not wanted and very distressful.

Frequently in our society we tend to undervalue the need for closeness, the time necessary and indispensable for "resonating" the sensations and behaviors of others; we prefer "doing" by ourselves and showing that we can do it instead of being friendly and warm.

We are clearly losing that way of staying side by side, that closeness that helps growth without forcing it and most of all that respect for the times and ways of a child and an adult.

I heard a beautiful sentence in a commercial of a charity dedicated to children in need: "listen to me when I am not talking!" In fact babies never talk, they act their emotions directly, if they are scared, sorry, angry, they do not use an immediately understandable language nor do they speak when asked. We need to be at their side; a parent needs to be intimate and welcoming.

If a mother is not warm enough at the beginning, the baby will retreat because her repeated rejections are too frustrating. The most drastic decision "for survival" might consist in reducing love offerings to the mother resulting in serious psychic conditions such as alexithymia, narcissism, psychopathology and paranoid states. The responses that will become more problematic with the passage of time and announce a future that will be affectively difficult for the child can be many and varied: the baby can look for love in an invading way and become clinging, or can opt for a safe distance, or fall ill often in order to receive at least material care, or become jealous and aggressive, possessive and destructive. Human beings cannot live apart; children need to find attention and recognition somehow.

Bowlby and collaborators (1988) showed that insecure attachment can create also responses that can favor autonomy: the baby pretends not to see the mother when she returns after a separation experienced as abandonment. But is that true autonomy?

How many persons today boast their "independence" from others, how many give to affective life only snippets of time, how many say they are happy with superficial, fleeting interchangeable encounters?

It is worth remembering how important others are for the construction of our identity, how important they are for supporting and maintaining our self-esteem and love for ourselves.

It is worth remembering that the ability of establishing affective relations with others allows us to be seen and valued for how we are: the deepest and most stable feeling of OKness cannot be reached and maintained for how we are seen and gratified superficially, for what we do or own but for what we truly are (Fromm, 1956).

Only the persons with whom we reach a certain level of intimacy can appreciate and know our true self, regardless of the social masks we usually wear.

The truly useful and indispensable feedback humans need are those exchanged in the truth of a relationship mutually deep, authentic and intimate that is not so easy to establish (Piccinino, 2012).

It is worth stressing that sharing and closeness to others are the only true resources that support out unstableness and finitude.

There is no medicine, or psychology, or religion, or philosophy, that can substitute the friendly hands that hug and comfort us in moments of fear, desperation, anxiety that inevitably happen in our life. An illness or even death can be better accepted when our loved ones gather around our bed. Their number and affection are the signal of the quality of our existence.

The attitude with which we face an illness is not only individual but also collective and the warm and kind participation of a community shows the relational quality of our life, popularity, warmth, dignity, humanity.

I am not talking here of passion or romantic love: in the fulfillment of the belonging drive what is at stake for us humans are closeness, intimacy, comfort, sharing and fondness of our existence.

To develop, protect, and consolidate the affective drive is the most important challenge to win for a human being, the sweet duty and the magical light that will illuminate and warm up a life.

## The most insidious and humiliating pain, not being able to evolve

One of the basic features of the system of "natural precursors" we are provided with from birth is that it is "self-feeding". I don't like this term, but I think it is explicative. I mean that human beings, once they get used to some happiness, not only tend to repeat it but suffer deeply if it ceases to be. This is true also in the case of other more ordinary and material needs, such as the quality of food or sex. In sum, if something turns out well and we are satisfied with it, we tend to repeat it all life long. But sooner or later we tire of everything, except of what is necessary and essential to our existence, that is, drives.

I repeat that we should not mistake happiness for pleasure; with the passing of time the latter becomes boring and is easily taken for granted unless it is somehow related to the emotional reward deriving from fulfilling a drive.

So sexual intercourse can be marvelous if it also fulfils an affective drive; otherwise after a while it becomes a mechanical act, not really pervasive, not really exciting, not really memorable.

Similarly, eating only rare delicacies can become boring in the long run if it is not accompanied by a discovery, social sharing or a need for survival, the latter three being again drive fulfilling behaviors.

In my personal ranking of the most memorable meals, for example, the best food for me has always been my mother's meatloaf, then the sandwiches eaten while chatting with my sister when we both were children sitting in the back seat of the car while our parents were driving us for a weekend outing, then a roasted fish prepared on a solitary beach in Cuba, shared with seven friends with one fork, and finally the first hot meal I had in New Delhi some 40 years ago after 25 days of traveling and eating just what I found. I still remember it was some type of meat and they called it Mona Lisa. But I feel the same when I eat ice cream with a sore throat or whatever food I have after a period of fasting or even "the first swig of beer" (Delerme, 1998) to quote a book on the little joys of life published years ago. The opposite example is the first dinner with my fiancée and her mother. I invited them in one of the most refined and expensive restaurants in Milan and neither of us remembered the next morning and remembers now what we ate.

Learning is an exciting impulse for humans; children soak in all kinds of information in the first years of life, always have their eyes and ears wide open, constantly ask questions, look for confirmations and try to learn more.

In a rhythm that is considered unbearable by an adult.

To explore, look around, ask, even try to guess, in sum, to get to know is the main sport of childhood, it ranks just behind cuddling. Children never tire, they want to learn and to structure in categories, they want to reach the condition of being able to decide on their own as fast as possible, they want to grow up by controlling knowledge, they want to evolve. They are perfectly aware that knowledge is power.

And as soon as they think they know something, they explain it to you, they use it to feel grown up and independent.

As it was obvious for our ancestors in caves, it is obvious for a child that knowledge allows them to choose better, to face the unknown in life with as few uncertainties and doubts as possible.

The more I know the world, the less what is unknown will also be threatening or dangerous; on the contrary it will be a moment of discovery and expansion. Through knowledge human beings have accepted, if not overcome, the fear of living, they stopped hiding during a storm and tried to understand what were those sudden bright lights that discharged on the ground and lit up fires. Knowledge gives joy; at times it excites or makes one proud, makes one feel a sense of fullness that elevates and brings one to a state of contemplative and spiritual wellbeing. To know and to recognize what is happening (within and without themselves) gives human beings a sense of peace and mastery of themselves and the environment that generates tranquility in the oddest and less comfortable situations. It gives mastery and force.

It is easy to see how important learning has been for the first humans and how important it is for a child or an adult facing the boundless knowledge one needs to live well. Be it a lot or a little, a child needs structure and stimuli, needs to prepare stabilized answers. Our minds need to categorize, collect, and organize a database stable enough to help us face the unknown, the sudden and the unexpected.

To learn means also to acquire in a more or less rigid way some patterns of behavior that exclude other patterns; it means also to "choose" quite early in what drives we intend to specialize. The happiness we will derive from this will be a reinforcement for those behaviors. So, almost unawares, we build values, practices, and habits, actual guidelines, that will accompany us throughout our lives determining many of our choices.

This is also the meaning of the term Script that, recovering and developing the old psychological concepts of repetition compulsion and self-fulfilling prophecy describes how the scenario of our life is determined quite early on by the outcome of our primary relations when our "wild and raw" nature starts to express itself and integrates with a Culture that should be "refined and evolved".

Returning to the drive to Evolution and Knowledge, let us remember that to grow, learn, discover and also teach and disseminate are opportunities that we all enjoy with great satisfaction at the beginning of our lives, and if they were guaranteed throughout it they could provide us with an extraordinary sense of vitality, power and usefulness. Evolutionism is within ourselves and for us like for all living beings, is a biological necessity consistent with the expansive process of the universe. But in this case too, if all goes well!

As for all our propensities, negative messages also in this case are the outcome of the more or less unconscious limitations and problems of our parents. It is rare to hear a mother or a father directly and willfully limiting the curiosity if their child. For this drive too limitations derive often by non-stimulating or indifferent or hasty attitudes or by an environment that is poor or scarce in knowledge. They usually are Injunctions to not thinking, not growing, not doing, that are the outcome of the Scripts of parents that find it hard to tolerate their child's vivacity and curiosity that request attention and availability.

In our societies there are still lively and strong trends to authoritarianism that devalue and mortify the exploration of patterns of behavior different from the usual ones, but if we are looking at early messages that inhibit this drive, it is rather a question of unconscious devaluations of the area of thinking and knowledge.

I think we can identify three wide problematic areas in parents that unconsciously tend to inhibit the drive to knowledge.

### Authoritarianism

The first area concerns very pragmatic and directive parents (in TA they are identified by the prevalent use of a Normative Negative Parent Ego State) that, being hardened in circumscribed, hyper-regulated lives and lacking stimuli, will tend inevitably to request predictability to their children: timetables, styles, self-expression, attitudes, and the like, will be strongly codified and regulated in an effort at reproducing exactly their personality and their codified worldviews. These are parents that do not intimately engage, their character armor is totally impervious to the novelty of their children's expressions, they do not acknowledge their children's personality and therefore constantly devalue them, especially from the point of view of autonomy. Frightened for themselves by freedom and lack of rules, they tend to respond to their children's "greedy" explorations in coercive and harassing ways.

### Possessiveness

The second area, similarly controlling and derived from the parents' insecurity, is instead affective and blackmailing and in general is the outcome of the fear of losing the children's love. This is why, being these mainly maternal attitudes, the parent establishes a pervasive and constant proximity that reassures her of her lovability and capacity. Very often this blackmailing and clinging hyper-affectivity (in TA these parents use mainly a Negative Affective Parent Ego State) is the outcome of traumatic breaks in the link experienced by the mother when she was a child or an adolescent. The old pain and the consequent fear of a present loss induce compliance and excessive care, a form of hyper-nourishment that overwhelms the child's needs and most of all inhibits their affective initiatives. The always invaded child will tend to surrender passively to the hugs, will suffer them but with the passage of time will not miss them and therefore will not desire them. The initial symbiosis will last too long favoring the retention of children in an infantile condition, hyper-protected and annihilating.

### Disconnection

The third area concerns a peculiar kind of abandonment, not necessarily material and affective, but rather existential, so to say. It is a distance that leaves the baby, and the child, alone with their own problems and conflicts, their own small and big difficulties. Lack of time, for example, haste and relevant engagements outside the home but also a certain idea of childhood (slightly archaic, I find) according to which "children grow by themselves", are all conditions favoring the child's loneliness. But also in this case I tend to consider these "explanations" superficial, covering deeper and unconscious lack of care, little intimacy, emotional disconnection. The mentioned material conditions are a very poor justification for personalities that are not quite available for healthy and appropriate parenting (in TA these behaviors are explained with a general lack of both the Affective and Normative Parent Ego State).

Parents that are still children, at times too busy with themselves, often with borderline or narcissistic personalities, distant because they do not know how to take care or play or wait silently for the "whys" and "hows". These parents, unable to walk along their child, putting themselves at their level of words and gestures, will end up inducing the same disconnection in their child too. The propensity to autonomy will be too early and too uninformed, lonely rather than independent, as we will see when discussing the propensity to self-assertion. Knowledge will be managed by the child alone with the more than understandable consequences of inadequacy and rigidity.

The conflict between the drive to grow/evolve/know and the inhibiting message can have different outcomes but there is no doubt that at six-to-eight months we can see some babies already happily exploring while others before any even short separation already turn imploringly or frightened to their mothers.

A very interesting study presented by a group of child psychotherapists at the mentioned congress in 2012, "Suffocate: strategies for survival", on the basis of video recordings made in the baby's home saw that the strongly asthmatic repeated responses of a baby aged a few months who had ended more than once in the hospital were determined by the excessive dedication of his mother who during the meals while lovingly feeding him with a spoon involuntarily prevented him from looking away from her. She called him to her all the time with endearments and a baby voice. That baby was literally out of breath, such was the dedication of his mother and the involuntary but asphyxiating control she exerted on him.

I mention this example to stress that at times the Injunctions (in this case they could be "don't be independent" and "don't go far", etc.) can reach the baby without intending to limit their growth. Simply (or tragically) the energy investment of the child on a drive or another derives from the inclinations (or problems) of their parent. In this case the propensities to exploration or autonomy had been sacrificed as compared to the drives to belonging and survival.

Obviously, it is not an episode that creates these Injunctions and the ensuing decrease in power of one propensity, but it is the persistent inhibition of the baby's actions in one of those areas.

It is therefore highly probable that if curiosity and exploration were qualities inhibited also to the parent and they will be experienced as a disruption when they powerfully emerge in the child and will be more often curbed than accepted with joy and enthusiasm.

I think that the pain for the curbing of the drive to knowledge is insidious because after all it is never experienced as a real tragedy. The baby needs certainties, craves for the repetition of fairy tales. Stability and calm in the face of an unknown and ever-changing world simplify life a lot.

So, mother's and father's assiduous closeness cannot but be experienced as salvation and resolution in countless cases as for example for avoiding the necessary pain of separation.

Unfortunately, in this way without realizing it the child will crumple, be contented, will become a "good child" adapted and subjugated, adequate to the surrounding environment.

When they grow these children will mainly choose stable and protective situations and environments, comfortable schools, sports, and friends where they feel welcome and recognized for their conformist personality.

So, they prepare and crystallize a flat and flimsy Script for life, without momentum, without risks, without the liveliness and curious initiative that is the salt of our existence at all ages. In this way they settle in an existence that is acritical, subjugated, afraid of what is new, grey, often prey of strong, protective stable personalities, necessarily normative and authoritarian. Suffering remains under the surface, silent, almost accepted as if it wasn't even possible to imagine a deviation from a path already set.

On the other hand, as I was saying, good submissive children are always very appreciated by their parents and by society and the sacrifice of evolutionary vitality receives an affective reward that is incalculable, at least in childhood: the love of mother and father is worth giving up diversity.

So many depressions appear surprising when they emerge in adulthood, when life suddenly seems meaningless, when a loss of stability and safety for the end of a love affair or of a job leaves the individual without the resources required to recover and start anew.

When repetitions, boredom, lack of stimuli mortify existence and self-value, even suicide can look like an exit strategy.

To imprison a living being like *Homo sapiens sapiens* is a mortal sin, a condition that goes against nature, the more so when the bars of the cage are only mental and an anonymous, a flimsy and bleak personality is faced with a world that is in constant evolution.

### The most corrosive and reifying pain, not being able to be oneself

The drive to differentiation that appears about three weeks after birth is usually a frank onset of diversification and opposition that challenges the patience and acceptance mainly of mothers. Suddenly the baby realizes with a surprise that is difficult to imagine that there is Another near them.

As I said, smiles are one of the first indulgent manifestations of love but immediately along with this demonstration of closeness, we see intense efforts at proving one's alterity. It is as if the baby wanted to show their individual existence to themselves and to their mothers; they have to show their right to diversity and, in fact, the assertion of their individuality is what favors one of the most important evolutionary shifts for the human species: the baby leaves symbiosis and undifferentiation and enters the world of intersubjectivity, of I-you.

This "innate you" ready to emerge meets an actual You, in flesh and blood, already well-structured, their mother. But what does a baby see when they finally "see" their mother? They see what Winnicott (1981, 1987) describes as the mother's response to seeing her child: surprise, joy, satisfaction, love, curiosity, or disappointment, indifference, rejection.

The perception of oneself, the perception of the world, the perception of what is an I-Other relation is established deeply and crucially in this period. It is as if a baby, who knows nothing about themselves and relations, for an odd magical event landed alone in a world totally unknown inhabited by totally unknown persons. The baby knows that there will be someone (innate I-You) but only when they meet will they have an idea of themselves, of that other and of the relationship they "must" establish. And that other is an omnipotent being from whom their existence depends; without the other the baby cannot live. Will the stranger be loving? Then I can be loving as well! Our relationship will be joyful and full of discoveries. Will the stranger be distrustful and grumpy? But then I am dangerous! Our relationship will be unbalanced, difficult. I will have to make myself loved, I will try to conquer their trust. Will the stranger reject me? But then I am not OK; I must be a nasty baby!

I will have to adjust, to obey, to do all they want. Will the stranger be at times benign and at times will they leave?

The history of psychology is full of interpretations on the outcomes of this encounter and the ones mentioned above are only a few hypotheses about the stabilization of the mother-baby relationship, therefore the beginning of a Script, but I think that there are countless possibilities and that to try to find general categories on which to base our work in the diagnostic phase and even more in the therapeutic one is counterproductive.

We can define many possible categories for the first maternal attitudes, but the children's responses are always very variable. From a practical point of view (for what is interesting for me as psychotherapist) the most important thing is to understand how the image of ourselves, of the Other and of the intersubjective relation has solidified and stabilized in time.

With the passage of years these images, or better these different consistent sets of opinions, values, behavioral decisions, aspirations, habits, usual emotions, and the like, stabilize, and confirm themselves until they become our reference and guiding systems for the various situations we are going to meet in our life.

The historical reconstructions that individuals make of their lives are extremely important for verifying the adequacy of infantile perceptions that, crystallized and repeated in the first years, seemed true and inevitable and are instead only the purview of a baby and the outcome of a "localized" repetition of attitudes and counter-reactions.

The point is that our Script, that is, the set of emotions, behaviors and opinions with which we face our life, has been built, as we have seen, by a baby on the basis of the encounter between natural drives and the messages related to them coming from those specific parents.

It should be necessary then to verify what came of it.

The relationship with the mother is obviously crucial for the formation of individuality and it would be truly odd if it were not so, given that a diversification implies a union from which to separate, an inside from which to come out, a symbiosis that needs to be ended.

This is why the mode of separation, always long and often difficult, once it becomes an experience will be part of a person's identity and of future ways to separate.

The model of belonging thus created (totalizing, hyper-loving, normative, ambivalent, good enough, etc.) for how it takes place should be considered an "a priori" to be dealt with by the drive to differentiation in order to realize the exit from the nest in the healthiest possible way. It is easy to think that a good primary attachment facilitates also a progressive and protected separation.

Differentiation and separation from the mother are the first fundamental steps of our self-realization, the urge to be ourselves, to make a unique, individual and unrepeatable opus of our existence.

Human beings seem to be the only living beings who have an individualizing proprioceptivity, the only ones who feel different, the only ones who know that a person's behavior is something different from what that person thinks.

Although many researchers are starting to see awareness of differentiation in families of dolphins, primates, and elephants, we still tend to consider animals as confused in their groups.

The fact of thinking independently from the herd has had, as I mentioned earlier, extraordinary consequences from an evolutionary point of view, such as different survival strategies, creativity, new inventions and research that at first sight seems pointless but at a closer look is aimed to wellbeing and safety.

The "no" a child says, their lies, small and large omissions, explorations, separations and returns, food preferences, and later in life fancies for other persons such as teachers, drastic and absolute choices, categorical judgments, and, in adolescence, manic expressions, extreme self-representations, individualized times, a peculiar sense of order, rooting for sports teams, music genres and later falling in love, career choices, vacations and friends, partners and, later on, the sense of their existence, the meaning of their profession, spirituality, and so forth, are all manifestations of a self-realization with which they personalize their existence, make it alive, energetic and enjoyable. If all goes well.

There is a positive family message, among many others, that can affect for better or for worse the enhancement of the drive to self-assertion: "You are important for me!"

Important in many ways, because I care for you as a person, as an individual different from myself, as a human being that is brought to the world not to keep me company, not to prove my value, not to extend my kin, not to guarantee a very private support in old age.

A human being is brought to the world to perpetuate the survival of the species in evolutionary, progressive, and improving terms; therefore it is nature itself that drives to autonomy in thoughts, actions, behaviors.

Parents who feel the importance of their children for the species raise them helping them to think with their own head, favoring the fulfilment of their goals, helping them to overcome difficulties with their own resources, give them a great permission: "you can be yourself!"

In this way a child will grow loving and thankful and at the same time independent to the extent that their parents have been able to accept their fancies and preferences, rejections and choices from the smallest and earliest ones that seem meaningless and instead are crucial for feeling that there is a permission to differentiate, to the grandest ones that will be adult choices aimed at fulfilling their talents and succeeding in life.

Injunctions and frustrations, in this case too, will be the more totalizing the earlier they are received and will crop up when the baby tries to get out of the symbiosis.

As we have seen with the asthmatic child, the prohibitions to autonomy are not always willful; in most cases they are considered protective while instead they represent a relevant devaluation of the child.

As always, if parents express messages of non-OKness ("You are not OK as you are"), children will "have" to adapt and surrender by accepting the limitations to being themselves "for the sake of survival".

Normally adaptations can be leaning toward submission when the child gives up their urge to autonomy, accepting strongly disciplined, restrained and controlled behaviors, or rebelling to the source of adaptation, the controlling parent.

Let us not forget, and this is why I call this pain "violent", that the healthy, original, and natural response to an invasion is anger, and the parental effort at limiting autonomy excessively is literally an invasion of the weaker by the stronger, is an abuse of power, is a constraint and in extreme cases a depersonalization against which one can only revolt.

The child adapts and submits, obviously if their surrender is somehow acknowledged, appreciated, and rewarded, but when this does not happen, then it is probable that they can only keep a total, provocative, counter-dependent, angry hostility or they choose a just as angry and resentful retreat, probably not so visible but ready to explode as a Rebel Child.

As always I am talking about early parental Injunctions that last in time. As proved by many cases I treated in my career, history (literally) is not made by solemn and exemplary prohibitions but by controls, suppressions, constant stifling, at times manipulating or strongly expressing a cultural consistency that makes the respect of the authority of the adult world seem totalizing.

One gets used to behaviors that are either compliant or rebellious and never allow one to feel what one truly would have wished had there been trust and respect for the child that even if young has inclinations and most of all dispositions of their own.

Children are born different, certainly not for the drives that move them that are universal, but for the strength and energy that they express.

Males are born male, psychologically, even when they are in female bodies, and females are born female even when they develop in a male body.

The level of aggression is different, biological gender differences are evident to any mother, female and male hormones with which children are born are variously distributed along a continuum where probably extremes do not even exist.

And therefore "Who am I raising?" should be the question that all parents should answer while carefully examining who they have in front of them. When starting from these premises raising a child can favor the expression of a specific and original identity: "You can be yourself!"

So, that child when they reach adulthood and for all their lives will feel important as themselves, an "aim" for themselves, never a means to fulfil someone else's aims, be they a parent, a spouse or even an employer and a community.

When they grow the persons that have received an inhibition of this drive will tend to know very little of their deep self, both on the depressive side (hyper-adapted children) and on the paranoid side (rebellious children); they will rarely be capable of truly "feeling" their needs and wishes and therefore to orient their life in a personal way.

Many of them can go on living modestly following the events, adhering to what is suggested to them by others.

Many of them can fill their lives with contrasts and skirmishes, always finding something or someone to blame for their inability to realize themselves. But all, deep down, will share the constant suspicion of not being able to live their lives.

Not many, unfortunately, come to therapy because they have perceived that their life is not very meaningful: the most adapted ones have such low aspirations that they never believe they can ask for something better to their existence and to themselves, while the angry ones, that very often are successful mastiffs, usually tell themselves they are OK only because, being quite active and energetic, they struggle and fuss in challenging and conflicting jobs.

The latter ones, that often appear like "winners" in this society, those who give the impression of being vital and living fully because of the speed and stress with which they live, those whose "not feeling" allows them to deny their solitude and mistake pleasure and success for the joy of living, these persons tend to wake up at a late age or because of some physical illness.

And it might be too late to reconsider the aims of their life.

It is ironic that in a culture like ours, more and more individualistic and celebrating personal success, many persons end up flattened in a meaningless and senseless life having forgotten that to be ourselves means first of all to realize our nature as human beings.

I present below a summary diagram where the Drives and archetypes are related to some examples of capacities that we can and should develop and realize.

| Survival | Belonging | Knowledge/Evolution | Self-Realization |
| --- | --- | --- | --- |
| EARTH | FIRE | WATER | AIR |
| Solidity | Affection | Curiosity | Creativity |
| Vitality | Kindness | Intelligence | Fantasy |
| Reliability | Solidarity | Critical mind | Intuition |
| Protection | Intimacy | Depth | Sense of self |
| Parenting | Trust | Listening | Vision of the future |
| Conservation | Sensuousness | Reflectivity | Autonomy |
| Perseverance | Amiability | Analyticity | Spirituality |
| Responsibility | Authenticity | Open-mindedness | Essentiality |
| Potency | Cooperativeness | Accuracy | Expressivity |

Those indicated below are the parents' adequate behaviors that favor their expression and realization and the necessary Permissions that must be experienced in therapy.

| Survival | Belonging | Knowledge/ Evolution | Self-Realization |
| --- | --- | --- | --- |
| EARTH | FIRE | WATER | AIR |
| Unconditional love | Unconditional love | Unconditional love | Unconditional love |
| Affective/Physical care | Empathy | Stimulus | Accept diversity |
| Thoughtfulness | Kindness | Protection | Protection from risks |
| Presence | Intimacy | Trust | Interdependence |
| Attention | Mirroring | Availability | Dialogue |
| Protection | Solidity | Backup | Spirituality |
| Potency | Spontaneity | Recognitions | Transcendent vision |
| Reliability | Containment | Curiosity | To let go |
| Responsibility | Physical contact | Encouragement | To stay |
| YOU CAN: | YOU CAN: | YOU CAN: | YOU CAN: |
| exist | love | grow | be yourself |
| be healthy | be intimate | think | be different |
| important | feel | evolve | be conflicting |
| vital | rejoice together | succeed | dream |
| mindful of yourself | cooperate | change | be spiritual |

In an article that I think was undervalued in the vast psychotherapeutic world, Fanita English (2008), one of the world's most important transactional analysts, in her article "What Motivates Resilience after Trauma?" mentioned three unconscious forces that constitute our psychic energy. She called them motivators, in total agreement with what I am discussing in this book. She described them as mysterious goddesses: "three goddesses, dancing high above us". Being a very creative and funny person, to explain their function she used funny and evocative names that have a classical echo "Survia", "Passia", and "Transcia".

If by Survia she intended the drive to individual survival (whose attributes are hunger, pain, the search for recognition and all that is necessary to keep us alive) and by Passia all the other motivations that activate the survival of the species (creativity, exploration, procreation, sexuality, courage, all the activations required for social life, etc. – I could say she groups here the drives of Belonging, Growth, and Self-Realization), with Transcia, and this is the most interesting aspect; she introduced a biological and existential need of human existence that has been constantly neglected. It is as if talking about breathing we mentioned only inspiration and forgot expiration.

With Transcia English described the motivation to get away from worldly cares, that need to let go, even the ability to relax, sleep, allow oneself passivity and idleness, the ability to let go and find peace even from an existential and spiritual point of view, in sum expiration.

She closed her article with the following slogans:

"From Survia: Take care! Here's to good health!
From Passia: Have fun! Enjoy! Here's to happiness!
From Transcia: Take it easy! Peace!"

In closing, a summary of pure and uncontaminated Human nature:

HUMAN NATURE IS:

For the Survival drive

ENERGETIC,   REPRODUCTIVE   PROTECTIVE,   DEFENSIVE,
AGGRESSIVE

For the Belonging drive

ALTRUISTIC, TRUSTWORTHY, COOPERATIVE, LOVING

For the Knowledge and Evolution drive

CURIOUS, EXPLORATIVE, HUNGRY FOR KNOWLEDGE, RATIONAL

For the self-realization drive

DIFFERENTIATED, INDIVIDUAL, SELF-CENTERED, SPIRITUAL

The features that describe the essence of human nature that should be defended or recovered are what I always keep in mind when I start on a path of evolution and change with a person. At times it is the finishing line, at others the starting point, but the awareness of which propensity is lacking is always a crucial passage in order to go on and develop together the relative abilities that had not been developed.

Even if they can help us identify the aims of therapy, our patterns and categories must remain only summary indications for the therapist: the names to give to Drives, Injunctions, Permissions and to the abilities will need to be identified by the patients; they must never be a diagnostic label pasted by the therapist, they should be the very personal discovery of one's limitations and the relative chance to evolve.

The "right" words, in fact, are only the ones that evoke in a person their ancient experience and that the person can acknowledge by saying: "Yes, this is it!"

Below a summary of the negative effects of not fulfilling drives.

---

### Inadequate propensity to Survival

Main emotional responses: ANGER with possible ensuing aggression and violence. Responses at times senseless and uncontrollable of attack and flight with paranoid thoughts or depressive withdrawal, catastrophic feelings. Frequent borderline syndromes and psychotic depersonalizations.

### Inadequate propensity to belonging

Main emotional responses: SADNESS and FEAR, even if not always identified and perceived as such, often one feels anxiety, distress, shame, sense of solitude or loss of identity. Responses at times paranoid and aggressive for the radical rejection of the Other but more often depressive isolation with self-harming behaviors or radical insensitivity and emotional de-sensibilization.

### Inadequate propensity to survival and evolution

Main emotional responses: SADNESS with loss of self-esteem and sense of one's value, boredom, uselessness, dissatisfaction, frustration, demotivation, mental rigidity. In general responses of resignation and mortification, depression mostly but with possible mythomania and sudden violence

### Inadequate propensity to self-realization

Main emotional responses: SADNESS with loss of interest for life, reduction in vitality, boredom, sense of emptiness, hollowness. Responses often depressively oriented with expressions of pessimism and superficiality. Cynicism as an effort at justifying and generalizing the lack of meaning and the emptiness of one's existence.

## Bibliography

Bollas C. (1982) On the relation to the self as an object. In *The International Journal of Psychoanalysis*, *63*(3): 347–359.

Borgna E. (2013) *La dignità ferita* (*The Wounded Dignity*). Milano, Feltrinelli.

Bowlby J. (1979) *The Making and Breaking of Affectional Bonds*. London, Routledge.

Bowlby J. (1988) *A Secure Base: Parent-Child Attachment and Healthy Human Development*. New York, Basic Books.

Brooks D. (2011) *The Social Animal: The Hidden Sources of Love, Character, and Achievement*. New York, Random House.

Delerme P. (1998) *La prima sorsata di birra*. (*The first swig of beer*). Milano, Frassinelli.

Diamond J. (2012) *The World until Yesterday: What Can We Learn from Traditional Societies?* London, Penguin Books.

English F. (2008) What Motivates Resilience After Trauma? In *TAJ*, 38(4): 343–351.

Fraiberg Selma H. (1999) *Il sostegno allo sviluppo* (*Development support*). Milano, Raffaello Cortina.

Fromm E. (1956) *The Art of Loving*, New York, Harper & Row.

Nowak M., Highfield R. (2011) *SuperCooperators: Altruism, Evolution, and Why We Need Each Other to Succeed*. New York, Free Press.

Orbecchi M. (2015) *Biologia dell'anima. Teoria dell'evoluzione e psicoterapia.* (*Biology of the Soul. Evolutionary Theory and Psychotherapy*). Torino, Bollati Boringhieri.

Piccinino G. (2012) La ferita dei non amaNti. (The wound of non-lovers). In *Neopsiche* N°12, Torino, Ananke.

Pievani T. (2014) *Evoluti e abbandonati*. (*Evolved and Abandoned*). Torino, Einaudi.

Sennet R. (2012) *Together: The Rituals, Pleasures and Politics of Cooperation*. London, Yale University Press.

Stern D. (1995) *Motherhood Constellation: A Unified View of Parent-Infant Psychotherapy*. New York. Routledge.

Tomasello M. (2014) *A Natural History of Human Thinking*. Cambridge, MA, Harvard University Press.

Winnicott D. W. (1987) *Babies and Their Mothers*. New York, Da Capo Press.

# Chapter 5

# The goals of psychotherapy, beyond emergency

Transactional Analysis has been one of the psychological schools that most focused on the idea that human beings are basically good, as, among the many, Rutger Bregman masterfully showed in his latest book *Humankind: A New History of Human Nature* (2019) (*De meeste mensen deugen. Een nieuwe geschiedenis van de mens*, 2019).

Eric Berne's focus on OKness as an essential feature of human beings and as relational mode for therapists and patients presented in his earliest writings (1947, 1961) has always attracted me and was one of the factors that made me choose Transactional Analysis as reference for my profession.

But, as I said at the beginning of the book, I felt something was missing and that the concept of Physis had not been examined thoroughly enough. For this reason, starting from the universal characteristics of all human beings as highlighted by historians and anthropologists, I found it necessary to discuss in depth how the endogenous drives typical of humans orient our lives.

They are neither needs nor hungers, but vital energy powerfully oriented to survival, love, knowledge, differentiation. In this sense also the need for recognition, stimulus, and structure outlined by Berne (1964) are not motivational drivers but conditions and messages necessary for the drives to be confirmed and oriented at their early onset and for all our lives.

We do not live to receive strokes even if they are indispensable, nor success or self-esteem, but to realize a biological project energetically oriented to survive, love, evolve, and realize ourselves.

Let us not mistake the goals of our life with the means to reach them; we are not so different from other living species.

Even a rose plant has to become a bush and like all other living beings is pushed by its initial form as seed from its very specific biological project to realize its nature: it will grow to a given structure, a given number of branches, a given height to make roses bloom and reproduce: it will have a specific continuity if it receives the required nourishment: the proper mix of sun, water and nourishment from the dirt. It will be hungry for that sun, water, temperature, and dirt and will search for that nourishment that we can call strokes, typical of its species.

DOI: 10.4324/9781003303831-5

So it will grow happy to bloom. Just like any animal baby and ourselves: blooming is the goal of humans too.

For this reason mental health and happiness are not only the consequence of a good psychic and relational functioning, nor of a good stroke economy, nor of being capable of intimacy and self-esteem, or even less of having reached one's goals and being a winner.

There's a lot more at stake: the realization of our nature!

In Transactional Analysis there is a clear awareness of this. For example, Berne in *A Layman's Guide to Psychiatry and Psychoanalysis* (1947) wrote about Physis: "there is something beyond all this – some force that drives people to grow, progress and do better". Fanita English with her "vital impetus" and her "Existential Pattern Therapy" (1976, 1988, 2008); Richard Erskine (2013) said "Physis is the source of our internal thrust to challenge acquiescence, to explore different ways of doing and being, to have aspirations, and to develop our full potential" (p. 6); and Carlo Moiso, in an article on the Script (1998), mentioned vital drives calling them "to be, to belong, to become".

As Bill Cornell reminds us (*Into TA: A Comprehensive Textbook on Transactional Analysis*, 2016), each human being has value and dignity and every baby is born with a basic existential position of OKness and will tend to *want* to realize it if environmental conditions favor it. Many other authors may have discussed this, but I feel that many TA scholars focused more on the good functioning of personality and on the importance of relations than on the essential characteristics of human nature.

It is not a question of deciding whether for human beings' natural drives are more important than relations, whether nature is more important than culture since they both are obviously important. It is a question of understanding how to make those natural precursors that were deteriorated in childhood reemerge and of bringing them to completion.

We therapists need to create a proper environment that like a new family can stimulate, welcome, and bring to completion these potentials once and for all.

There is no doubt that psychotherapy must always answer the patient's requests and that disorders are often serious. Anxiety, depression, borderline syndromes, but also more common symptoms such as anorgasmia, premature ejaculation, anorexia/bulimia, panic, phobias, and the like, often require immediate interventions aimed at reducing the state of distress as fast as possible.

This is the reason of the importance of the technical knowledge that allows us to face immediately and with competence and efficacy any catastrophic or melancholic experiences, but in this book I am presenting that part of therapeutic work aimed at the "big target", a radical and definitive change, for what is possible obviously, with a specific person at a specific age.

I do not forget that great distress is always accompanied by devastating material situations, but although we often have to provide "first aid", we must never forget that human suffering is always what I defined as a mismatch of nature and culture, of what our drives and our nature expect for us and what the initial years of our lives have allowed us to fulfill.

If we want to be happy when we become adults, we need to secure what of natural and essential we did not receive as children (the fulfilment of our propensities).

In the summary schemas I presented at the end of the previous chapter we can see the abilities that persons with little drive energy in a given area had to forgo; it is evident that different drives refer to different areas so that one can be well "equipped" to fulfill a drive but totally unable to fulfill another.

For example, if a child received early Permissions to know and explore, they will usually also receive the abilities required to become a champion in that direction; vice versa, if the propensity to belonging was stemmed by brusque and rejecting messages, it will be difficult to grow with the ability to be intimate, trusting, open to relations and links, etc.

Two considerations derive from this:

• On one side, a generalized OKness does not always exist. In most cases people are truly realized and satisfied in an area and unexpressed in another also because the messages mothers and fathers send are often quite different and addressed to different areas.
• On the other, during therapy we have to keep account of the fact that if a person has become aware of the lack of development of one drive, they will also become capable of giving themselves relevant Permissions, even if they finally "decide" to develop that new part of themselves, they need to keep account of the fact that they are beginners, dilettantes, neophytes in that internal and external world. In order to acquire that ability, they need a lot of training, discipline, continuity and "assisted" experimentation.

There are no such things as miracles or shortcuts in human change. Emotional success, rebirth, energy received from above or from pyramids of light, revelations on family history, cannot but deceive and disappoint; in most cases these phenomena upset a person with useless "annunciations". The human mind must restructure itself deeply in various neuronal areas for a change to take place.

We should therefore talk of more or less relevant problems and distress, more or less early inhibitions of nature, short or long term goals, work aimed at reducing distress or at evolving that person's Script and their personality structure.

A serious and deep understanding of the intervention required, diagnosis in short, is necessarily an awareness reached together while respecting the cognitive and emotional possibilities of the patient.

Psychotherapy is a path of progressive knowledge and discovery; there are few certainties we can cling to, even the drive map, the concepts of Script, Injunctions and Permissions and all the rest, are basically the attribution of a general name to events that are not general at all: each person will have to identify the permission for their specific prohibition, will need to reconstruct their history from what they think happened, from residual resources but with the certainty that what is typical of human nature, however buried and unused, will always be recoverable, at least in part.

We will then have to discover the rest, a new healthy and positive part of the Script that we will formulate and verify together. From then on we too will have to use those terms we identified in the path together and forget our terms. So we will no longer talk of depression, phobias, injunctions, manic defenses, and the like. We will stop interpreting and surprising patients with our wonderful intuitions and will start instead to see together what actually happened.

We will find the proper terms, those the patient considers as most appropriate to describe their story and their feelings and we will do it, as much as possible, with the gaze of two (or more if we are a group) adults at the same level.

The aims of therapy should be identified, declared, and decided together (Berne, 1966), just as we understand and decide together when to end treatment and why. Patients can stop when they want, obviously, even if it will always be the therapist's, the doctor's, task and responsibility to choose what to say at the end, even to inform about the degree of "humanity" (health) reached.

I mean that to make patients responsible for the course of the therapy does not mean to cancel our professional position.

What I question of many psychotherapies is that in some cases in the final phase of treatment therapists feel relieved of their responsibility on the life of a person who asked them for help. Not to share my perplexity and preoccupations seems to me a bashfulness out of place, a secrecy that represents a default of help and presence when a very relevant choice has to be made and, like all separations, can be another topical moment to analyze.

Imagine that a repair technician did not signal the presence of rust in your car even if you just brought it to check the engine or fix a tire and did not recommend the proper maintenance actions and good driving practices. This would be just as irresponsible.

What people do in their life is just as important as what happens in sessions and a therapist should take care of that too. Life too must change if we don't want to leave a person in the same situations they encountered when their knowledge was limited and they came to us for help.

To change oneself means also to change one's life.

Forgive my frankness, but cold and detached persons live reasonably well because they move often and establish cold, detached and superficial human relations.

Similarly, psychopathic managers of big companies are surrounded by faithful dogs and can remain impervious to the suffering of the workers they exploit and lay off (see on this Jon Ronson's "The Psychopath Test"). – the depressed too, as long as they have someone taking care of them, and so on.

What I question of many psychotherapists is the lack of global responsibility for the persons they talk to: we do not treat segments or parts of people.

We simply help them to recover a natural and healthy life walking with them in their discovery of themselves, widening their opportunities, a journey that inevitably becomes also our journey.

We psychotherapists are not and will never be perfect, for sure, but we have the responsibility of embodying at least the wish and the effort to be healthy and aware of the path that each human being should walk to give value to their existence and be happy.

We must be the first to have a healthy and happy life and a great relational sensitivity.

But there's another crucial question that "divides" the world of psychotherapists: can we change without analyzing the past and making it emerge?

Alice Miller wrote: in "*The Drama of the Gifted Child: The Search for the True Self*. Completely revised and updated with a new afterword by the author" (1997):

It is one of the turning points in therapy when the patient comes to the emotional insight that all the love she has captured with so much effort and self-denial was not meant for her as she really was, that the admiration for her beauty and achievements was aimed at this beauty and these achievements and not at the child herself.

(p. 14)

This means it was addressed to him turning into a Adapted Submissive Child, we would say.

The abuses Miller saw in her professional life show that evil lies precisely in the inevitable negative use (*ab use*) that the parents make of their children to "satisfy" themselves.

Not only sexually, but more frequently to fulfill through their children their own need for success, links, self-realization, financial safety, happiness. All these are abuses!

And when this happens, the life of that child will no longer follow its natural course, oriented to fulfilling not their own drives but those of their parents. Their life will be directed to give fulfillment to the previous frustrations of their parents.

The "deviated" child in the end will believe to be so from birth, to have been born that way, and will tend to accept this condition as natural.

This is why to discover that many of their limits, difficulties, sufferings *do not* depend on themselves is a crucial message at the beginning of treatment, an awareness that is in my opinion inevitable if they want to go further and take up their responsibility for their present life. Can we change a person without freeing them from the suspicion that their unhappiness depends on them? And Miller adds:

> If a person is able, during this long process, to experience the reality that he was never loved as a child for what he was but was instead needed and exploited for his achievements, success, and good qualities – and that he sacrificed his childhood for this form of love – he will be very deeply shaken, but one day he will feel the desire to end these efforts. He will discover in himself a need to live according to his true self and no longer be forced to earn "love" that always leaves him empty-handed, since it is given to his false self – something he has begun to identify and relinquish.
>
> (p. 60)

And I totally agree; I have had the very same experience with patients coming from other therapies. To change a behavior is relatively easy and sometimes fast if the sacrifice of our natural drives has not been induced deeply in the first years of life."

Which means in short that that person is already basically sane.

Alice Miller did not really believe in "pardoning the parents" and had many a reason to criticize those therapists that press patients to a premature pardon inspired by religious values.

I met many persons that believed they were at peace with the past only because they had "understood" the problems of their parents.

Pardon is not healing (as we will see in depth in the chapter "The Basic Fault is the Wound of the Non-Lovers") if the feelings of pain, anger, even hate nursed all life long have not emerged.

We must first let them emerge from the unconscious and express them and be aware that it is right to feel them. The child part of a person must not be silenced again as it happened in childhood; on the contrary, in many cases they should be pressed and pushed to be finally able to be angry and therefore to differentiate. At the time fear was huge, and today for many it is just as difficult to respond to rejections, abuse and injustice.

But even the liberation of aggression is not healing; as Berne would say, it only "make[s] them braver frogs" or angry frogs. The ambition of this book is precisely to go beyond "seeing and understanding truth"; in my opinion we need more; we need to learn to love the world as it is and ourselves in it, in a natural and evolutionary view.

A last consideration on the drive system is that few will not have seen that the four drives integrate among themselves and in couples that can seem but are not one the opposite of the other: survival/conservation on one side and knowledge/evolution on the other. But one without the other becomes a prison, a dangerous and frustrating sentence. They must never be in antithesis nor unbalanced; they are all inevitable biological needs for a human being. On the other hand, I think it is clear that we can explore only if we are anchored to our strong roots; we can be creative and find new inventions only with the support of an array of previously accumulated knowledge.

Ulysses could "follow virtue and knowledge" because at home he had Penelope and his son Telemachus that "held" the kingdom. A bit too comfortable to tell the truth but functional to the war task he had assigned to himself and that we imagine was temporary (because we are benevolent). But when his throne and riches we in danger, even Ulysses, the famous wanderer, fought with all his strength to recover them.

Without a safe base an explorer is only foolhardy, his courage is recklessness. To fly away one always needs a base well rooted in the mind that provides the safety of conservation and survival.

One can think of the rest when the expansive evolutionary drive is developed, the one that lets us out of the nest because in nature all living beings guarantee their survival through more or less deep, frequent, evident interchanges with their environment.

Similarly, belonging and self-assertion seem to be located on opposite poles, and in fact different psychological problems end up located in this polarization: on one side the symbiotic, on the other the narcissistic, but we know very well that in a healthy and natural development, both drives must be present and active.

We are always engaged in it because life itself invites us to invest our energy in different drive areas in the various stages of our life.

In adolescence in all cultures a very strong need for independence from the family emerges but to be able to separate, youths must at the same time join peer groups where they can build new links, stronger than the original ones, with new different values, at least apparently, but enough to be able to say, "I am looking for my way!" A new belonging often becomes necessary for reaching autonomy from a previous relation.

If the four drives have been welcomed in childhood, the propensity to express them equably and the abilities required to fulfill them will be always alive and sound in our Script, even if in some periods of life one can be stronger than the others. So one can be able to travel around the world with a solid affective background, well protected by an internalized passion for life.

Similarly, we can establish tight and lasting links without fearing losing a fragile and shaky individuality.

Similarly in an adult a real and deep autonomy is possible if there is also soundness and trust in oneself, internal safety, self-protection, and most of all that feeling of quiet and peace that is formed only with a positive parental contact in childhood that allows us to feel that one can fall but without falling to pieces.

A truly autonomous person knows how to ask for help, knows that when their personal abilities prove insufficient, and it happens (it does!), they will find someone to help them.

So belonging without autonomy becomes dependence from a "dominating other", as in depressed persons, while on the contrary autonomy without belonging ends up leading to isolation and loneliness, as in cold and detached persons.

When brought to the extreme each drive takes all the space at the expense of the others and becomes our reason for success but at the same time our pathology.

We need balance and harmony between propensities, a true miracle of accord of sounds that only the awareness of our deepest nature and our ability in guiding our life can help us realize.

In order to extricate ourselves from this tangle of urges and experiences, we really need an exceptional emotional and reflective competence, an overall view, a long-term view, and at the same time exceptional attention to the here and now.

I think the goal of a good psychotherapy is to help people to be happy or better to be able to reach happiness by harmoniously fulfilling all their drives, first of all the love drive that requires an extraordinary capacity of offering oneself and loving the world and people just as they are.

Usually this means to restart the propensities frustrated in childhood because what we have not learned to fulfill as children we have to learn to do as adults.

If we want to be "good enough" human beings.

## Bibliography

Berne E. (1947) *The Mind in Action. A Layman's Guide to Psychiatry and Psychoanalisys*. New York, Simon and Schuster.

Berne E. (1961) *TA in Psychotherapy*. New York, Grove Press.

Berne E. (1964) *Games People Play*. New York, Grove Press.

Berne E. (1966) *Principles of Group Treatment*. New York, Oxford University Press.

Bregman R. (2019) *De meeste mensen deugen: een nieuwe geschiedenis van de mens (Humankind: A Hopeful History)*. Amsterdam, De Correspondent BV.

Cornell W. F., De Graaf A., Newton T., Thunissen M. (2016) *Into TA. A Comprehensive Textbook on Transactional Analysis*. London, Karnac Book.

English F. (1976) Racketeering. In *Transactional Analysis Journal*, 6(1): 76–81.

English F. (1988) Whither script? In *Transactional Analysis Journal*, 18(4): 294–303.

English F. (2008) What Motivates Resilience After Trauma? In *TAJ*, 38(4): 343–351.

Erskine R. G. (2013) Vulnerability, authenticity and inter-subjective contact: Philosophical principles of integrative psychotherapy. In *International Journal of Integrative Psychotherapy*, 2: 1–9.

Miller A. (1997) *The Drama of the Gifted Child: The Search for the True Self. Completely Revised and Updated With a New Afterword by the Author*. New York, Harper Collins.

Moiso C. (1998) Being and belonging. In *Script*, 28(9): 1–7.

Ronson J. (2012) *The Psychopath Test: A Journey Through the Madness Industry*. New York, Riverhead Books.

# Chapter 6

# Life scripts between drives and adaptations

We barely reflect on this, but we must admit that a growing child with their bursting vitality and naturality disrupts their parents' modes of life, habits, values, their Scripts in sum, if they are a couple, harmonized, properly balanced, and stable, "accommodated" in a daily humdrum.

Their personalities are "settled" and each of them has more or less realized propensities, a more or less fragile OKness, adaptations, modes of managing time, individual and couple identity.

Obviously if they are fairly happy and realized, they will welcome their newborn looking at their extreme behaviors and bossiness with affection and indulgence, they will know how to answer the requests, dampen the exaggerations, contain the dramas, accept some rejections denying others with measure and joy.

Unlike the newborn for whom everything is new and who has only one priority, to be accepted to survive, the parents should already have been living for years in a well-protected and already stable balance.

They have plenty to lose in front of a human being that is totally Natural and loud in their expressions, the more so if they are blocked in limited personalities and have given up the realization of some of their potential. They have many certainties to lose.

In other words, the baby, that is Natural by nature (inevitable repetition) literally slams in the face of their parents their limited scripts and the negative choices they must have made while building their identity.

Take for example my father, who was a stern person and developed a habit of respectfulness from a life of submission. How do you think he could have responded to his Child stating: "I don't want peas, they are awful!" and later on "You can't understand, you are old!" See what we considered daring at the time as compared to today's adolescents.

We tend to imagine a fragile child at the mercy of their parents but if we look more closely quite often we see the parents at the mercy of their little tyrant.

DOI: 10.4324/9781003303831-6

But this applies also to a deeper level: not only the parents are often overwhelmed by their child's "arrogance" and power but are also challenged by their wild and powerful nature, strongly alternative to their lifestyle.

Let's think of the baby's attachment drive and how with cuddles and hugs the child impacts their mother's affective mode, her usual warmth and physical closeness, and how this reaches the father and elicits jealousy in some cases and engagement and participation in others. Or how it elicits disapproval and disgust for a so-called gush expressed so shamelessly.

The Natural Child is the Self of Human Nature (Sills and Hargaden, 2002) that is faced with the "false self", character armor, Ego and Script, consolidated and stiff personality structure of their parents.

It is as if a naked child, like the happy boys that we sometimes see on the beach, met another child dressed up in a suit and tie. One of the two would feel out of place and inadequate. But which one? The newborn who knows nothing or the one already beloved for dressing up like a little man?

I think it is now time to understand these parents better, and I would start with a couple of considerations that I find important for explaining their fragility. The first one concerns the lifestyles they are often forced to "wear" and pass on to their children, while the second one refers in particular to the problems mothers face when they become pregnant.

We adults are all fossilized (to different degrees);, we cannot deny we are all the outcome of a long struggle between nature and culture (in the sense I explained previously) and each one of us stabilized on more or less pervasive and stiff adaptations.

In TA these adaptations have been studied and called Drivers (Kahler, T. 2008), a term I don't like very much because it is too generic and can be given many other meanings. I prefer to call them "lifestyles" or "adaptation styles" to denote a mode, a pattern of behavior that is repeated and used to be accepted and welcome as children and as adults at the beginning from our parents, later on from all others. And in the end, and as a consequence, also by ourselves.

Once consolidated these patterns are "justified" by our own value systems. Once settled in our daily life they become a sort of Ego offered to the others as a business card introducing our social acceptability.

But let's proceed step by step.

We adults have been children and according to how our "natural precursors" have been received, we will have felt more or less OK, loved, and welcome.

But when a parent (who in turn has been a child, has had parents and so on) devalues a drive, usually they not only devalue it but also offer an acceptable alternative.

"You cannot do that; do as I say" – this is more or less the essential and immediate language of a parent irritated by the presence of a child that overturns their existence while "I am not OK as I am; I am the wrong one" is the translation that the child makes when these messages are repeated.

We see below, analyzing each drive separately, how frustrating messages can induce unhealthy and unnatural behaviors and what can be the new beliefs that need to be analyzed and changed in treatment.

## Survival

How can a baby survive if they "perceive" messages that make them feel unwanted or that they are being neglected, rejected, and abandoned to themselves or are not important for their parents? What can they invent and learn to do to be accepted or at least welcome, if they do not feel loved for what they are and their very right to existence is questioned?

And a mother or father who does not take care promptly, does not have enough time or interest for the baby's existence, what will they say, how will they justify their little care? What model of life will they offer? We can imagine this kind of exchange: "We accept you *if* … you are independent, strong, autonomous, if you grow fast and don't ask for too much, if you show us you can do without us".

The functioning models suggested to the child will become their way to avoid feeling the deep anxiety caused by that early abandonment, by that "You are not Ok" or "We don't want you", a sort of "Do not count on us too much" that is unbearable.

The child will have to protect themselves by becoming first of all a STRONG child or one that cannot remain a child, needs to grow fast, not lean on others, without fancies or gushes or tantrums, what we call HURRY UP. Or they can become PERFECT, a child and later an adult that cannot afford mistakes, is able to do everything perfectly on their own, cannot show limitations, difficulties and negative aspects of themselves.

In all these cases, with the different features typical of each of these lifestyles, the obvious consequences will be the typical behaviors of those who have not had time to be children but had to become adults too fast: you cannot ask for help, your needs are not important.

You have to be the best, never show inefficiency, you must earn recognition and acceptance through doing and showing (more or less obsessively compulsively) your value.

The trouble is that a person will look for recognition and attention based on those typical behaviors, losing sight of the fact that self-esteem and self-assurance become rooted only through unconditioned acceptance and not through behaviors that obsessively look for confirmations of one's actions. Praise for actions will never dispel the doubt that one is not OK as a person, nor can it protect from the fear that if one day one is not able to fulfill those expectations, the suspended anxiety will emerge along with the horrible suspicion of "not being OK".

When I was a child there was an inflatable rubber doll, as tall as a child, that one could punch and hit but always got back up on its basis. It was called

Ercolinosempreinpiedi (Always-up-on-your-feet). When you are invited to BE STRONG, you have to be always like that: never collapse, never bend. It is evident that these behaviors, strength and rapidity of action and indestructibility, can be easily rewarded and confirmed with satisfaction by parents that are afraid of fragility and of the intrinsic weakness of children.

No sane parent would ever say openly (but I heard some say it half-jokingly) "I don't want you" or "damned be the day of your birth" or "I don't care about you" or even "I wanted to have an abortion but my parents insisted and ..." but if it actually happened or if a parent thought it, the child will perceive it from their off-putting attitudes, will understand it from sentences like: "stop whining for nothing" or "I am not going to wait for you to be ready" or even "you are ruining my life".

The messages that question the child's OKness come through in a million ways and, given the very long time children and parents spend together, we see that they can be very hard-hitting, given also the state of objective inability and uncertainty that is part of everyone's childhood. At the same time, it will be very easy to specialize and repeat always that typical "style" because those parents and the whole world will praise it and its outcomes.

That child will grow strong and defended, stiff and unforgiving with themselves and others. They will lock in a steel armor any fear, uncertainty, fragility, doubts, and a sullen suspicion, the distressing impression of being a bluff, of not being OK, of being totally wrong. So they will not be able to get near their fragility because this would immediately evoke the fear they started avoiding as babies with the help of that STRONG behavior.

So when they become parents they certainly will not like their children's tears or tantrums, they will feel troubled and hostile toward those childish behaviors.

Their children's fragility will irritate them, forcing them to face their own internal prohibitions, their denied behaviors, reminding them that in their childhood sanctions were associated to "if you do that, I will not love you".

This is the struggle I was mentioning above between the bursting vitality and naturalness of a Natural "drive" Child and the parents' lifestyles, now rigid and consolidated.

Parents always think they are teaching a style for the "children's own good"; they are surely teaching what they thought was the "secret of their success in life".

This is what therapy needs to discover: how those behaviors were only the secret of those parents, their Script, their model of life, and the reference values from which they chose their behaviors.

The STRONG ones, but also the others, will have to re-discover how they sentenced themselves to those behaviors to be accepted by their parents, who in turn were dominated by that same style. They will have to re-discover their human traits of fragility, doubt, uncertainty and most of all that today, unlike in their childhood, they can be lovable as they "naturally" were, re-experiencing with the new people they meet how they can be important, acceptable and at the center of their own existence, persons that can be loved deeply.

For SURVIVAL the most important Permissions to achieve are:

You can be as you are, you can exist, you can be in the world and be healthy, you can be important and vital, you can take care of yourself and your material and psychological needs, you can take care of and protect your environment.

## Belonging

Many adults when they become parents show a relational coldness that not even their adoring and depending child is able to dent. At times the mother's and father's stream of love that is always present in the first months (Ammaniti M. e Gallese V., 2014) rapidly deflates because too often the jobs of both partners prevail on the newborn's needs.

When the relation that provides a safe base is broken too early and suddenly, the baby perceives that an unexplainable catastrophe is taking place. The baby cannot let the symbiosis dissolve slowly with its natural times while their propensity to autonomy emerges. It is something coming from the outside that interrupts the idyll, often without respecting the baby's natural rhythms and progressive distancing.

Even we adults are inconsolable for a long time when a love affair is suddenly dissolved. Imagine what happens to children who have no idea of why it happened and if there can be someone else in the future.

We must also remember that these early separations always leave a mark, even when they are well offset by good adoptions or warm grandparents. I remember a patient who had a very warm relation with her father until she was about seven or eight; at that time her physical warmth scared her father, who perceived it as sexual and therefore dangerous and reacted with a drastic and total separation from her that the girl unconsciously thought was her fault because she was growing up and becoming a woman. She tried to recover the relation but failed and considered this as her father's contempt of her, so she became totally cold and stopped any motion, any expression of love, and any offer of intimacy to him.

She therefore condemned herself to total isolation that lasted until one day in therapy she was able to attribute a different meaning to that separation: it was not her that had done something wrong, it was her father who was scared. When she understood this, she finally concluded: "Poor dad, how scared he must have felt for his own sexuality!" She progressively reactivated the wish to have new warm relations.

In my work I met many mothers who complained of their cold children but seeing them there in front of my desk or in a group, so cold and detached or so normative, I was not surprised at all.

As I already said, if a child backs away when their love is frustrated, they are protecting themselves by remaining alone, avoiding contact, retreating in an individual and solitary world where there is no room for any "illusion" of love. Those fragile parents unaware of their own coldness could easily conclude: "What can I do; my child has always been cold, they were cold from the start".

Bowlby and collaborators (1979, 1988) wrote extensively on this and also about what they call an ambivalent mother, the one who takes care when she needs it and becomes more invasive and protective when she has time and when she feels guilty for her many absences.

A child cannot but take a position of "independence", of defensive detachment that has nothing to do with the acquisition of autonomy because to reach autonomy one always has to overcome dependence, not do without it.

A child becomes autonomous when the dissolution of symbiosis is the outcome of a process that accepts and favors the child's first attempts accompanied by mother and father in total safety, not an unexpected or early banishment from heaven.

Alberto Torre, one of my supervisors, often reminds me that "for a child their mother is the world, for an adult the world becomes their mother!" Dramatic?

We learn with the mothers that at the beginning are all we have but then we repeat what we have learnt with others, as if they were our mothers.

The most frequent adaptive response is the HURRY UP driver that will make us disinvest not from human relations but from feeling truly and deeply engaged in a love relation. There is such a fear to "depend" on a person – "that surely later will leave me" – that we prefer to live moving from one relation to another without ever stopping. These persons are very good at establishing fleeting and little engaging relations, even great romances, provided they don't last long and always leave a way for escaping.

Speed, independence, efficiency will be their great qualities, and they will also be valued for them, but feeling totally engaged in a mature relation open to the future will be perceived as a trap, an illusion for silly, romantic persons, an impossible fancy for insecure and needy personalities.

At times an adaptation style deriving from this disinvestment in the family can lead us to try to be acceptable, showing abilities, so the child will try to be the best child possible, both in terms of BE STRONG and BE PERFECT, depending on where praise was directed, more to control, power, and solidity or to efficiency, precision, excellence.

Sometimes it will be possible to produce stable attachments, but the mode will remain far from intimate, loving, warm, deep, with consequences also at the sexual level as the body has remained too long stone cold, insensitive, not willing to let go trustingly.

There will be anorgasmia, premature ejaculation, excessive promiscuity, and the like.

When these children become adults the relations with their children will be experienced as too engaging, as a loss of autonomy that prevents the free expression of their individuality.

It will not necessarily become a rejection, even if children will often experience it as such, but the fear of feeling again the pain of separation when it comes. Because the catastrophic fantasy will always be: "Sooner or later I will be set aside and the other will leave".

I know persons that prefer to go to the hospital alone, even for big surgeries, rather than show themselves as needy or not up to the dazzling fitness they tend to display in order to look OK.

Their relation to the therapist will be just as feeble at the beginning; they will not always come to sessions and they will be often late; when in a group they will find it difficult to open up but it will be the unveiling of their fear of the link with the therapist or the group that will represent the door to access their previous story of abandonment.

Often we hear of parents that lost their parents when they were very young, dramatic stories that left them desolate and without the force necessary for a new affective investment – stories of deep loneliness where coldness was only one of the many efforts at avoiding further pain.

We will have to go and "track down" the scared child and take them out of their loneliness and make them try what a new love relation can be.

From then on it will be possible, with great patience and respect for their mistrust, to start again with the therapist and the group the symbiotic relation that had been interrupted with their mother: first attachment, first enjoying to be trusting, first offering affective riches, first the creation of a safe base for unconditional acceptance and then, when the drive to autonomy will resurface, let the giddiness of separation and the joy of returning home slowly and gradually develop.

Persons must successfully experience more than once (and this is why treatments need to be relatively long) their right to wish for closeness as well as separation: "I can love, I can wish to leave, I can form a link, I can even depend and then if things go wrong I can feel free to go".

I insist that the drive for autonomy must always coexist with the drive to belonging.

For BELONGING the most important Permissions to achieve are:

You can love and be intimate, you can feel closeness and enjoy together, you can rely and trust, you can let go in another's arms, you can cooperate and remain autonomous, you can depend and love as you can separate and go.

## Knowledge/evolution

What kind of parent can a person who feels threatened by a child's wish for knowledge and growth become? Who can respond by trying to dam and suppress this drive?

The answer is at the same time easy and complex. Frankly I am not sure that they are a generalizable category but one trait they have in common is a stiff character that prevents them from accepting favorably that enthusiasm for knowledge that looks for explanations for everything and explores the world in the most unthought of directions. Enthusiasm.

I like to repeat that this word derives from the Greek "en theos", a God inside, a God that activates, moves, energizes, expands with a vital powerful cognitive force that we all have inside.

A child in the first years of life must learn millions of notions, their minds light up, feed and add up every piece of information. Every day the knowledge drive leads them to store thousands of notions, every day for months and years, pushes them to seize as fast as possible all the tools they will need to live.

A child is a force of nature that sparks off questions, explorations, doubts, criticism, competition, all attitudes that challenge parents with fragile personalities, little self-esteem, who need to find in their child a confirmation of themselves rather than a challenge. Insecure parents find themselves in front of a little smart guy that looks for certainties and cannot wait to outdo mom and dad, a little explorer who literally hard presses especially those hyper-protective mothers who are afraid of their own autonomy.

A person's insecurity is the fiercest enemy of knowledge.

Many parents have children to have a confirmation of their OKness, to be reassured of their own value, to be finally able to impose themselves on someone else.

They like easy wins, having someone now to guide, indoctrinate, control, bring up in their own image. Persons that were dominated by their family of origin now become lions within the walls of their home. How many children (and how many women) find themselves related to this kind of men, weak with the strong and strong with the weak, competitive, full of resentment for what they suffered in the past, ready to engage with their children in useless and tiring skirmishes or even epic battles on who knows best, who has more right to define life and the world. Or who has to hold the remote control! "Don't do what you wish, do as I say!" "Where do you think you are going without me?" "What do you think you know?"

If this little polymorph (certainly not perverse) explorer does not feel accepted as they are, what can they do to be accepted but TRY HARD to follow in their parents' footsteps, if their evolutionary energy turns out to be so dangerous. What can they do but give up their passions, their inclinations and prove their worth following the paths indicated and trodden by others?

PLEASE the adult will be another way to obtain recognition and esteem, once again the simplest and most immediate way to avoid the fear of rejection, to feel accepted and finally see their parents satisfied with them.

The fuel of knowledge is passion; personal choices activate intuition and creativity, certainly not adaptation to what others think is good for us and even less the sense of duty. The message children often extract when their enthusiasm is thwarted is "I am nothing special, but if I try to do what they suggest, if I do my best to reach it, then they will be happy of me".

Insecure parents are often unable to be happy and enthusiastic when they see in their children's eyes the blazing light of curiosity, of intelligence, of possible "genius".

So they end up sentencing their children to the mediocrity of a narrow Script limited to a familiar horizon.

Even on the female front, hyper-protective mothers, more or less ambivalent or invasive, hinder the development of their children's potential with their constant presence.

Terrorized by the possible losses that they probably suffered, often unawares, these mothers tie their children to themselves with an enveloping net of care and exaggerated protection. By mediocrity I don't mean to stress that these persons will end up being or feeling like losers; they will simply have little faith in themselves and if they succeed they will do so vicariously, joining other people's projects, making do with much less than they could have.

They will not necessarily be less rational or brilliant, they will only be little self-centered, little capable of asking themselves: "What do I really want to do with my life? "How do I want to be?"

They will be good support hands, very good deputies, great workers but without too many whims.

They will always be a little envious of the success of others, especially when they realize that those with a habit of feeling capable will not have their same need to engage as much as possible to do what they want.

The typical adaptations will lead them to TRY HARD to achieve tasks set by others, to show their huge engagement; since they don't think they are brilliant, they are never able to stop even when it is clear that what there are doing is not what they are made for.

Their priority is to show that they try hard until they are exhausted: "Look Mummy, look Daddy, how I try to do what you want". In this sense it is also a way to learn to PLEASE.

In both cases one gives up growth, evolution, fathoming various alternatives, discovering the world, being active and reflective, analytical, critical, and most of all trusting one's own abilities and possibilities.

The frustrated drive is that to evolve but also the one concerning self-realization that implies a good differentiation and the ability to live one's life as one wants.

For KNOWLEDGE/EVOLUTION the most important Permissions to achieve are:

You can grow and think with your own head, you can succeed doing what is good for you, you can change course if you realize the course you are on is not the right one, you can be different from how others want you, you can be as you are and like yourself as you are.

## Self-Realization

This drive is activated for the first time in the process of differentiation in those extraordinary moments when the newborn actually "sees" the Other for the first time, separating from the primeval union that until then had been container and content, a concept that is even hard to think. To be human beings without an Ego!

But this seems to be the condition of almost all living species: they don't know they are individuals. Human beings instead separate perceptively from their mothers about two or three weeks after coming out of her body. I try not to call birth that moment.

The time needed for being born is much longer or we could more correctly say "My birth is when I say you", which is the opening line of a beautiful poem by Aldo Capitini (1956).

That moment is always celebrated also because mothers suddenly realize that something sensational has happened.

The newborn smiles and looks for her face, wants to touch her deeply in love and enthusiastic, shows a different attachment and slowly but pretty soon starts opposing and doing what they want. The concept of self-realization is much more comprehensive than that of differentiation because in the subsequent years this "natural precursor" will evolve in more complex directions as the child starts asking questions prompted by their feeling different from others and having a reflective mind.

But let us return to the question of the struggle between nature and culture, between the Natural Child and parenting. What will happen if this propensity, that is so unique among all living beings, is opposed and thwarted?

What psychological state affects the parent that sees the autonomy and difference of their child as a danger for them or for the child? It is not just a normal and understandable difficulty in identifying in the child, even more so if the child is of the opposite sex; here I am talking of fragility, deep fear, unconscious responses.

I take examples from the stories told me by persons that were reflecting on their difficulty in being themselves.

The message, the request of adaptation that often the parents send can mainly be included in the PLEASE ME style but can be expressed in different ways and derives from different problems experienced by the parents.

The fear of separation, for example, plays a very important role also for this drive, especially for some mothers who tend to create excessively tight and warm links. They fill their children with attentions, they are always available, they indulge them in everything, they turn them into the love of their life. The more they are frustrated by their marital relation, the more they choose their child, preferably a boy, but not necessarily, as partner of an idealized relation where the age difference plays strongly in favor of a "patronizing" attitude.

Years of frustrations, of early separations from their attachment figures, of submission, of physical exertion, of acute distress can be offset by a new relationship where they are from the very beginning queens and uncontested mistresses.

"No woman will ever love you like I do!" is a statement that often can slip out and become the threat of the "good" witch that is however convinced of reassuring the child on the eternity and indissolubility of their love and in this way makes them her slave.

These needy mothers unconsciously ask their children to solve their problem of symbiotic attachment, protecting them from the pain of even the earliest brief separations. The child will not be happy to go to kindergarten and will easily capitulate when they see their mother's sad and distressed face. Every NO will almost be a tragedy, every "I don't like it" will receive disappointed responses, and so on.

Obviously, the role of fathers in these situations can be very important both in confirming the tendency to keep the child in the family or, on the contrary, in re-establishing the marital couple thus favoring the progressive exit from symbiosis. A mature link should be based on parity, mutual respect, love, and autonomy.

In the past few years we have seen more and more clearly that many males find it hard to accept the rejection and separation from the woman they love; frequent violent episodes tragically show that too often their identity depends on the presence of an exclusive and unconditioned romantic relation.

But in addition to sociological and cultural considerations, we should reflect and try to understand that in many cases those same men have been "brought up" by families that poured on them a possessive and totalizing love. We should reflect on why adult men cannot stand on their own, cannot bear to be left and consider owning a woman their "existential quality". The problem is how they have been taught to love.

Those parents, even many mothers, will have involuntarily erected and idolized a totem to a masculinity to which all is due and that can claim everything. Our male chauvinist culture infiltrates and often still defines the relations between parents and children.

Each case is different but certainly those children do not learn to feel OK without that link and, at the same time, having received too much dedication, will never be able to question their "narcissism". The others never understand, they do not love enough as compared to the love these persons provide and consider limitless and total, just like the love they received as children.

The drive to adaptation can be superficially an apparent and sometimes sweet PLEASE ME, but below the surface there will be the anger and aggression of a person who had everything from a relation.

A "macho" must prove to be more than a strong master in the very moment he feels he is losing the love that made him feel omnipotent, without actually being it, and at the same time feels he is falling in a terribly feared fragility.

As years pass the drive to self-realization forces us to face a series of existential issues that are suggested by the reflective capacity of human beings: "What am I doing here?", for example, and "What am I doing of this life, what is it for, who am I, what happens after death?"

Questions that children ask and that will come back in mature age more unavoidable and pressing to question our intelligence and sensitivity.

Life is a sense-less folly for us humans when it has no "sense", no aim or direction. We must find a meaning to avoid that sense of sadness and emptiness that seizes us when we feel we lived in vain and we did not fulfill our talents and potentials.

This is why one of the highest aims of psychotherapy is to help people to ask these questions and find "their own" answer.

It is neither philosophy nor religion; it is addressing the drive to realization just like we addressed the other drives. And the drive to self-realization "imposes" to us humans, provided of individuality free will, reflectivity, to realize what our condition of privilege and responsibility suggests to us.

It is a privilege to be born human beings and a responsibility to have the power to co-create a little universe, were it only our little personal garden.

We will go back to this because the joy we can obtain from the realization of ourselves is probably the most intense and satisfying, is that sense of fullness, that joy of living that includes having been able to also fulfill the other drives: to have survived, to have reproduced, to have loved, to have evolved.

The persons who have not developed this drive often don't ask any questions; they live, how can I say it, by chance, following heterodirected paths of life; they consume their lives as they consume what is suggested by the media, as if those objects or lifestyles were essential while they have little in common with happiness. Thinking autonomously for them is difficult just like feeling to be in deep contact with their own originality and uniqueness.

With the therapist they will have to walk again the path that was blocked in childhood and at last establish a link that gives them value as individuals, capable of developing their own direction in life.

For SELF-REALIZATION the most important Permissions to achieve are:

You can be yourself and be different from others (including the therapist, obviously), you can have conflicts without necessarily cutting links, you can feel what you feel and think with your head, you can leave and live alone, you can value your existence as a Good that you can realize.

A summary scheme

| Drive | Adaptation styles | Permissions to achieve in therapy aims |
|---|---|---|
| TO SURVIVE | BE STRONG BE PERFECT HURRY UP | You can be as you are, you can exist, you can be in the world and be healthy, you can be important, vital, you can take care of yourself |
| TO BELONG | HURRY UP BE PERFECT BE STRONG | You can love and be intimate, you can feel closeness and enjoy it together, you can rely and trust, you can cooperate and remain autonomous, you can be intimate but also separate |
| TO KNOW/ EVOLVE | TRY HARD PLEASE ME HURRY UP | You can grow and succeed in life doing what you prefer, you can change course if you realize the course you are on is not the right one, you can be different from how others want you and like yourself as you are |
| TO SELF- REALIZE | PLEASE ME HURRY UP | You can be yourself and be different from others, you can feel what you feel and realize your talents and your identity, you can give direction, meaning and value to your existence and leave a positive mark on your passing |

In closing this chapter, I think I need to clarify some concepts.

First of all, the adaptations, that, as I said, in TA are called Drivers, here are described rather briefly. Whoever wants to know more about them can find a comprehensive description in my book *The Joy of Working* (Piccinino, 2006), where I also included a questionnaire to facilitate a diagnosis.

I mention it here because in therapy I often start from these observations that are usually quite visible in behaviors so that I can then go on to Permissions and the abilities the patients need to develop to fulfill the relevant drives.

I already said more than once that to reactivate our "natural precursors" is for me the essence and often the final aim, when possible, of treatment. And this is why even in the scheme above I included first the arrival drives, then the adaptations that hamper our nature and in closing the Permissions required as a means to reactivate the drives.

I think is useful to highlight a second warning that, even if I already mentioned it, these systematizations make use of generic and synthetic words and are used by therapists to reflect on the features of the person coming for help and on the probable course of the treatment.

In the sessions we will then have to find together the most meaningful descriptions for each patient, digging up their parents' voices and implicit messages and their indications to be accepted.

Parents can have told their children to be obedient and sensible, to never give up, to be reliable, secure, independent, a good little guy or a sweet little girl. In short, each person had their ways to meet their parents' requests. The adaptations can have been followed by the child in a more or less obsessive way, depending on how early they were imposed, but most of all on how much the parents were afraid that their child would not be OK *without* those specific behaviors.

Except in very rare cases, for me it is evident that parents always want to teach their children how to live well. In this sense love is implicit and granted, at least in their intentions.

But it's their fragility, fears, manias, paranoias, and obsessions, the conclusions they have drawn from their lives, that make the parents "instill" also violently their lifestyles in their children.

We will have to question their ways, not their love; it is by identifying the parents' prevailing styles and by understanding their motives that we can recover their love.

This is why I don't like to give a constantly negative view of the adaptations received, because they also represent qualities that can be useful in life, the more so when they are no longer an obsessive duty but one of the various options available.

To be resistant (STRONG), precise (PERFECT), fast (HURRY UP), persistent (TRY HARD) or compliant (PLEASE ME) is not wrong as Petruska Clarkson (1992), Julie Hay (2009) and Cornell, De Graaf, Newton and Thunissen (2016) made very clear. It becomes wrong when my acceptability, lovability, self-esteem and OKness depend from that indisputable behavior.

On the other hand, until I can accept and shamelessly show also the other side of the coin, my hidden shadow, I can't be sure that I am lovable as myself *with* my flaws and limitations.

Armors, false selves, adaptations are a sentence to non-authenticity with the underlying terror of revealing a bluff.

Also, the attribution of each drive to an area of the adaptation style should be seen just as an example since the variations of behaviors that derive from a drive are many, and each person "manages" in their own way when they are devalued, and much will depend on the life examples that the child will have seen around them.

In many cases the presence of grandparents and other relatives, for example, can fully offset the parents' idiosyncrasies for a given drive and make a given DRIVER less inflexible.

I am thinking of a couple of independent-thinking and free-behaving grandparents who were an extraordinary example for their granddaughter, although her parents openly and repeatedly condemned her autonomy. At the beginning drives are acted by children with force and without filters, their nature is enhanced and activated. If they find an even minimal chance for expression, we can be sure they'll profit from it, that light will attract their little flame because it will confirm that what they feel coming from inside themselves is not as wrong as other adults are trying to prove.

I know of teachers who disproved the negative prophecies of parents made distrustful by life and developed and respected the drive to knowledge and autonomy of students that had been depressed and turned off by too many devaluations.

And it was my personal experience too.

And I saw therapists blow lightly on a fire and saw their patient's joy of life and love shine brightly under its light.

At times a little is enough, at others, we need years, at others we don't really manage to do it, but human nature has been the same for millions of years and it passed through inquisitions and false prophets, destroyed books, saints and heretics burned at the stake, sexophobic and male-chauvinist religions, nihilist philosophers and bad teachers and obviously also limited psychologies and pedagogies.

Human nature, as I tried to prove in the first chapters, has been much stronger than all this. I trust that, as soon as it can, the true self of human nature always emerges. At times we just need to see where the fire is and blow on it.

Sills and Hargaden wrote (2012):

> We feel therefore that it is wholly appropriate to locate the self in the Child. ... Moreover, a theory of self is necessary to the methodology we propose, which involves the psychotherapist in using his or her "self" to bring about change. A central premise of the model is that elements of an undeveloped or disturbed early self emerge in the transference within the client–therapist relationship and that the transferential relationship is the major vehicle for deconfusion.

In other words, therapeutic work is based on separating (de-confusion) the natural true self (drives) from the adaptations that reduced, distorted, or modified them.

Adult and parental capacities, mental faculties, knowledge, abilities, scientific discoveries, technologies, the whole culture that the child will learn to know while growing must be at the service of that self.

## Bibliography

Ammaniti M., Gallese V. (2014) *The Birth of Intersubjectivity. Psychodynamic, Neurobiology, and Self.* New York, W. W. Norton & Co.

Bowlby J. (1979) *The Making and Breaking of Affectional Bonds.* London, Routledge.

Bowlby J. (1988) *A Secure Base: Parent-Child Attachment and Healthy Human Development.* New York, Basic Books.

Capitini A. (1956) *Colloquio corale* (*Choral Conversation*). Pisa, Pacini Mariotti.

Clarkson P. (1992) Physis in transactional analysis. In *Transactional Analysis Journal*, 22: 202–209.

Cornell W. F., De Graaf A., Newton T., Thunissen M. (2016) *Into TA. A Comprehensive Textbook on Transactional Analysis*. London, Karnac Book.

Hay J. (2009) *Working It Out at Work; Understanding Attitudes and Building Relationships*. Watfoord, UK, Sherwood.

Kahler T. (2008) *The Process Therapy Model: The Six Personality Types with Adaptations*. Little Rock, AK, Taibi Kahler Associates.

Piccinino G. (2006) *Il piacere di lavorare* (*The Pleasure of Working*). Trento, Erickson.

Sills C., Hargaden H. (2002) *Transactional Analysis. A Relational Perspective*. London, Routledge.

# Chapter 7

# Primary love and the ambivalence of mothers

I opened this book by talking about my father in order to emphasize how much our childhood experiences in the family are influenced by impressions and experiences that are always subjective.

But this is all the more true if we refer to mothers who are from many points of view almost always the most important figures for emotional growth. The depth, intensity, frequency, and therefore the quality and duration, of the relationship with mothers, from the earliest days of gestation and then in the first months of life, become as a matter of course, crucial for adequately accommodating the infant's first spurts of attachment. Yet of these days the child has, despite the fact that its life is greatly influenced by it, an intermittent, limited and often altered memory (Alberini and Travaglia, 2017).

Mothers then in the Western world are more and more alone in dealing with child care. According to the Washington-based Pew Research Center, in the whole world, the United States has the highest number of single parents: 23% out of total households according to the latest available data (2018).

According to this study, in fact, almost a quarter of US children/young people under the age of 18 live in a family with only one parent, usually the mother.

In Great Britain it is 19% while the European average is 13%.
(Source: Eurostat https://ec.europa.eu/eurostat/statistics-explained/
index and https://www.truenumbers.it/famiglia/monogenitoriale)

Italy, in this sad ranking, is in the sixth place, single parent households are 15.8% of the total and of these 86.4% are made up of single women.
(Source: Istat, Indagine sulle strutture e i comportamenti
familiari, Rome, Istat, 1985)

A dreadfully heavy job for these women – first hormones overrun their behavior, forcing them to a task required by the species, then they must manage the various heavy tasks with less and less support from their families that at least in the near past used to be around with a joyous and protective attitude.

Nowadays mothers tend to be alone in doing their job, and in the West they are even more alone because they are often single. But it is not just the exertion,

DOI: 10.4324/9781003303831-7

the sleepless nights, the responsibilities, the exhaustion, still quite undervalued in our cultures, to affect how they welcome a baby, but rather their adaptation styles, as we have seen, and their internal conflicts.

It is inevitable that women in this delicate phase of their life are caught in a frank ambivalence in a state of great psychic and physical stress.

Umberto Galimberti wrote on the Italian daily *La republica* on December 9, 2006:

> In women, in fact, more clearly than in males, there is a struggle between two antithetic subjectivities as one lives at the expense of the other. A subjectivity says "I" and another that makes the woman feel a "repository of the species". The conflict between these two subjectivities is at the basis of maternal love, but also of maternal hatred because, as Sophie Marinopulos (2005) reminds us, a child, any child, lives on and feeds of the sacrifice of their mothers: a sacrifice of her time, her body, her space, her sleep, her relations, her job, her career, her loves other than the love for her child.
>
> (Source: https://ricerca.repubblica.it/repubblica/archivio/
> repubblica/2006/12/09/dalla-parte-delle-madri.html)

We should add that often the distress of the perinatal phase is not perceived by the mothers and by the persons around them; very often is even denied for shame or guilt.

Winnicott (1987) was the first to expose the 18 "hates" of mothers toward their children and to accept them with a sense of understanding and "pietas".

Children are not interested in this but perhaps when these children grow into adults (and their therapists, who have been children too), they must build themselves a more realistic view, for this reason maybe we side with the mothers.

These are in fact real problems, not "fancies" or "hates" or "manias", not even that evident and understandable exhaustion that is often assimilated, generalized and labeled as post-partum depression: a psychological state that deserves a less generic and less dismissive consideration with greater attention to the individual situations that could very well explain its onset.

Childbirth is always a watershed for both parents, but for women it becomes a true test of drive balance, stability of identity and propensity to attachment.

In the following scheme, I tried to summarize the problems mothers can meet in this very delicate developmental phase where different needs and requirements, requests and expectations from the outside, objective difficulties, internal conflicts between being self-centered and hetero-centered, meet.

Let me add that often for the good luck of many newborns, the five ambivalences manifest themselves mainly when mothers realize that their child is not exactly as they imagined them, therefore not in the first months of life.

I suggest that what is remembered as a strongly negative attitude was often preceded by a good, if temporary, safe base that at least in part helps to avoid worse psychological consequences.

Below find a summary of the internal conflicts that mother will probably meet and would require a careful listening and an adequate support to be accepted, faced and overcome.

| Maternal Ambivalences | |
|---|---|
| TAKES UP THE ROLE OF PARENT | REMAINS CHILD OR ADULT |
| Is generous, available, solid | Is needy, voluble, self-centered |
| CHILDREN ARE WANTED | MATERNITY IS SUFFERED |
| Is altruistic, responsible, warm | Is revengeful, passive, disinterested |
| CHILDREN ARE ACCEPTED AS THEY ARE | CHILDREN ARE REJECTED FOR WHAT THEY ARE |
| Is joyful. accepting, exciting | Is devaluing, detached, abandoning |
| SIDES WITH CHILDREN | SIDES WITH THE REQUESTS OF OTHERS |
| Gives value to diversity, gives the right individual value, welcomes specificities | Is subject to the expectations of the families of origin, interprets the wishes of others on the role and character of children |
| LETS GO | RETAINS |
| Allows autonomy, can find the right distance, favors separation when the child goes | Is symbiotic, hyper-protective, hampering, experiences separations with anxiety and conveys preoccupation |

As I said, if it is true that the mother's mind changes in a way that strongly enhances loving parental attitudes to reach true devotion and care that become a source of happiness for her (Ammaniti and Gallese, 2014); it is also true that this happens to a person with an already well-rooted personality and a defined Script on her way to become a mother in a totally peculiar way.

The passage from the condition of woman to that of mother, especially in the case of the first child, is very delicate and forces upon her such a radical change of personality that it challenges her very identity and body image.

It is an existential change of role, of material condition: first she is female, young, independent, responsible only for herself, an adult that can also be a child, openly needy, voluble, self-centered but also free, self-assured, insouciant, independent, sexually active, in work, and so forth.

But often, even without great advance and preparation, comes the forced passage to altruism, to the preoccupation for the future, her own and that of her child, to total availability to the other, to the sacrifice of herself, the transfiguration of her body image and shape, the loss of sex appeal and often also of excitation.

And it is not necessarily a change that happens at the first maternity; sometimes it is even more difficult if a child arrives when she is older or by chance or when she is too young.

However beautiful, natural and desirable maternity is, these changes produce very personal responses in women.

How many certainties based on beauty, independence, freedom become drastically limited? And how do women react, with what feeling of rejection, sadness, rebellion to this kind of slavery to which they may be unprepared and especially little understood and supported?

Galimberti adds in the same newspaper article above:

> It is here that the love-hate ambivalence, well known to the mothers more than the fathers, becomes powerful and needs a solution that cannot be found but in recognition and acceptance of this ambivalence as natural and not in the guilt that can derive from interpreting it as a flaw or inadequacy of feeling.

Or worse by interpreting it as true and deep hatred toward her own child!

It is also a political problem because I am convinced too that first industrialization and emigration with the ensuing uprooting of family couples from their social environment, then the incredible growth of economic needs, have pushed many women to find a hurried job and maybe also to devalue the role of mother and distracted society as a whole from a delicate reproductive task that from time immemorial has required the engagement of a lovingly united community.

Mothers today are psychologically more and more alone and their "fragility", despite our increased psychological knowledge, is often enhanced by the requests coming from themselves and from society.

The stories of persons coming to psychotherapy, when they are able to look at their past with a less angry look, are full of stories of early, unwanted, unaware, superficial maternity, distracted by extra-family jobs.

At times it seems a miracle that given their conditions of rejection, abandonment, ignorance or violence, these mothers with these fathers have however been able to take care of their children in a way that if not adequate has been at least sufficient to avoid inducing more serious psychosis.

For each of the dyads I described in the scheme above we can suggest what psychological problems can arise.

| TAKES UP THE ROLE OF PARENT | REMAINS CHILD OR ADULT |
|---|---|
| Is generous, available, sound | Is needy, voluble, self-centered |

If the mother remains a child, she can easily make excessive behavioral requests to her child so that the child becomes her adult parent, she can induce them to take care of her or of any siblings with the consequence of inducing a Rescuer Script that will be applied also in adult age in taking care of others (PLEASE ME). Her child must not give reasons for worry (BE STRONG) because mother is too busy with her own worries. Her child will have to grow up earlier and faster than normal (HURRY UP).

So that child will be a master at autonomy, will easily fulfill the safety and evolution (knowledge drives, partially the belonging drive but will certainly find It hard to think of themselves and try to realize themselves).

| CHILDREN ARE WANTED | MATERNITY IS SUFFERED |
| --- | --- |
| Is altruistic, responsible, warm | Is revengeful, passive, disinterested |

When maternity is suffered, there might be frequent anger attacks, affective blackmailing, resentful criticism toward the child that will obviously feel they are the cause of mother's "sacrifice" as she is forced to take care of a child she did not truly want.

The child could turn away, feeling unwelcome and not feeling closeness, tending in turn the aggressive or hyperactive behaviors used to try to attract mother's attention into a character structure.

They could activate mutual psychological games of Victim/Persecutor where both end up feeling victims of abuse or of the other's excessive requests.

The most probable Drivers for the children will be BE STRONG, TRY HARD, and HURRY UP to try to offset the impossibility of experiencing a belonging relation.

The children who feel rejected are those who will more easily feel they are not OK and will suffer for a lack of self-esteem and safe base.

In any case, total rejection of children is rather rare since the mother's body (and her mind too) change independently from the condition she is in when she becomes pregnant.

In most cases rejection kicks in after a few months when breastfeeding, mirroring, the dance of gaze and smiles, has already taken place and therefore the psychological damage, although dramatic, can surprisingly end up not being totally pathological.

| CHILDREN ARE ACCEPTED AS THEY ARE | CHILDREN ARE REJECTED FOR WHAT THEY ARE |
| --- | --- |
| Is joyful. accepting, exciting | Is devaluing, detached, abandoning |

In this ambivalence, much depends on the seriousness of the rejection.

As I already said, it is rare that a parent says openly "don't be yourself" or "don't be intimate" or even less "don't be male (or female)" but will rather use expressions that disparage the qualifies underlying those behaviors, applying the attitude they disparage to their child's behaviors. So they might say "don't be stubborn; you are conceited", "don't be this sticky; you are clammy" or "don't be so gross and violent" or "don't be so gushy".

The children's distance from the parents' expectations, especially when large, is always a trauma for the parents, the more so if a family is nuclear and lives in a situation where the culture is one way only and strictly applied.

In such cases it is almost inevitable that such messages are internalized by the children as normal and plausible.

They will probably be in the area of BE STRONG, or PLEASE ME but also HURRY UP with more detailed attributions like be more feminine, more aggressive or more humble, more altruistic.

From this purview, as Galimberti also noticed, Western extended families in the past and the current ones in countries where there are more natural extended situations (I refer again to Diamond, 2012) offer to children a much larger array of possibilities, in TA terms, much less rigid and univocal Scripts. The parents' "manias" and obsessions can be more easily diluted and toned down by the messages of other members of the community.

| SIDES WITH CHILDREN | SIDES WITH THE REQUESTS OF OTHERS |
|---|---|
| Gives value to diversity, gives the right individual value, welcomes specificities | Is subject to the expectations of the families of origin, interprets the wishes of others on the role and character of children |

If we observe this ambivalence from a sociological point of view, unlike in the preceding case, here the Western world offers less danger of homologation; today's families, that used to be actual dynasties, tend to influence new couples, less so because they make up their own culture and also because they travel within countries and around the world.

In these situations the opposed risk is more frequent: children are moved around places already when very young.

As we know, children need safety and a solid affective and material structure, protective, foreseeable, even in the sense of a "safe base" that avoids confusion, the lack of continuing relations, the uncertainty of too much learning in relation to the child's age.

However, in the work I make with couples (that I usually perform in a couple with a colleague) I saw quite often sealed family Scripts where the fate of children was already marked from the grandparents down, even independent of (or even against) the mother's expectations, as she in turn had subjected to them.

The mother can be caught in between, often alone, and has to find a difficult balance between the child's right to be themselves and the external pressures that they expect from her, and therefore from the child too, the continuation of family culture.

If the mother succeeds in finding a balance between the belonging and the self-realization drives, she will also be able to defend her own pedagogical and psychological choices, while instead, if she is confused with her past and entangled in the family history, she will orient her child to be how their respective families expect, conveying the message TRY HARD to be like grandmother or become a doctor like your father or become a great man like your grandfather.

The risk is that, if she is not fully convinced of this choice, the mother, or the father, sends more or less unawares, contradictory messages that stimulate confusion and scarce conviction. We must not forget that a self-image forms on the mirrorings of parents and the damage is always a more or less evident and early conflict between natural propensities and environmental requests.

If the child received balanced Permissions in childhood, it will always be possible to change course; the world is full of persons that have been brought up strictly but then took different courses.

But the Permission must have been given, even if not too openly.

I remember a beautiful movie, *Dialogue avec mon jardinier*, directed by Jean Becker in 2007, where a successful painter wondered why he had been able to become an artist although his father had always opposed him and had prepared for him a safe and healthy future in his village chemist shop. But after his father's death, the painter finds in the attic some beautiful drawings made by his father. He is really surprised because he had never suspected that his father might have had a flair for art as he had always fought his son's inclinations. The movie does not say it explicitly but with his discovery the painter understands that his father had put aside his passion because he felt compelled first of all to provide for his family and ensure to his son a safe and comfortable future by sacrificing his own artistic inclinations that did not provide as much comfort as the chemist shop.

The second is that probably the son's passion for art had somehow been transmitted, even indirectly, through his father's thousands of contemplative attitudes, attention to nature, attention to details.

Children very often realize their parents dreams, even if not fully expressed; to see a frustrated mother or a father sacrificing his life is for a child is an indelible lesson, just like seeing their eyes shine or their commotion when contemplating an aspiration that has been frustrated by the material priorities of their generous lives.

If they had the permission to do it, children will not follow their parents' road even if laid in gold.

| LETS GO | RETAINS |
| --- | --- |
| Allows autonomy, can find the right distance, favors separation when the child goes | Is symbiotic, hyper-protective, hampering, experiences separations with anxiety and conveys preoccupation |

We must always remember that the initial symbiosis is totally natural and that mothers develop various hormones for this, even the five senses and some mental faculties become enhanced, like hearing, for example, so that mothers can hear their child's crying even when covered by other noises or understand the request the baby makes only based on their inflection and tone of voice.

Even separation is a natural process accompanied by neuronal changes, but these are fragile hormones (like oxytocin) easily affected by the subject's character, or so it seems.

We are therefore talking of developmental phases where a balancing factor should kick in: mother's happiness independent of her relation to her children.

A loving couple relation where she receives love and recognition, feels realized not only as a mother but also as a person, will keep her away from the temptation to cling to the lifeline of this relationship for receiving love, esteem and consideration and at the same time will free the child from the responsibility of being the one who makes mother happy.

It is not, as many say without realizing the sense of possession implied in the terms they use, of "having a child" but of "bringing a child to life", and there's a great difference!

And there is a great difference in bringing children to the world *because* one is happy and bringing them to the world in order to be happy.

The inevitable ambivalence of being a woman and a mother can be overcome "according to nature" if there is marital happiness and if the woman finds a proper balance between the belonging and survival drives that privilege the mother/child relation and the self-realization and evolution drives that orient to separation.

The healthy symbiosis of the first year loosens progressively according to nature under the emerging pull of differentiation and growth of both mother and child and also that of the father, who wants his partner back and, the same time, if he too takes care of the child, frees the mother.

From the point of view of the memories of one's past we could divide roughly the persons coming for therapy into two groups: the elusive and the angry.

The first ones tell themselves and tell us the story of a normal childhood without great problems, "like everyone else", they add and usually they don't know what happened.

I saw, although I don't have a proper statistical record, that these persons have all had ambivalent mothers who alternated abandoning attitudes with overwhelming and invasive closeness.

For these persons it is very difficult to hold on to resentful memories considering that their mother was often warm and caring.

At the same time it is ambivalence that elicits in children a certain diffidence and detachment that leads them to not experience (and therefore not remember) a particularly joyful relation of which one can be proud even when this actually happened, although in the way I described.

Therapeutic intervention with them is aimed at letting the memories and the complexity of responses emerge in order to stir their emotional apathy and help them recover the control of their affections.

The angry ones, instead, already know everything, remember all the injustice they suffered, the wrongs, violence, abandonment, they spend hours detailing the flaws of one or both parents; they know very well who is to blame and how these "misfortunes" befell them.

With them, as we will see in the last chapters, we will always have to fight these monsters and witches, the ogre parents that these patients keep alive and working within themselves.

They are true champions of blasting the Red Cross, so we will have to focus on recovering a more plausible and understandable recollection of what happened.

On the other hand, a child frustrated in their natural drives could not but actively defend themselves and explain to themselves what was going on with easy tales of witches and dragons eating children, as we all tell.

Ogres actually exist, but in reality they are persons that have become evil and confused and, most of all, often unable to establish acceptable loving relations, even with a child.

Once the child has found an explanation for their distress, they end up interpreting everything in the same way and, rather understandably, they forget all that does not fit in this general view.

Father then will be the good guy and mother the bad guy (or vice versa), a brother will be the parents' favorite while they are worth nothing because they were not wanted, as is totally clear. Men are all selfish as mother says (or vice versa), and so on.

This is why I think it is important that all therapists keep an empathic accepting position toward patients but without taking for granted that the situations they report are thorough and objective. Closeness and understanding must be directed to distress, rage, and fear, not necessarily to reported events.

If treatment wants to achieve a deep and stable change, we very often need our patients to revisit the story of their childhood, and of their parents and report it also to themselves in a new way. It can be a painful to unveil it, but in the end it brings solace, peace, and joy, but most of all love.

Making patients understand the fragility of parents and of mothers helps to highlight what they were not able see and to understand when already as children they had sewn on themselves a Script and had given themselves a dramatic explanation of the world: they have been loved by parents who were fragile, unbalanced, distressed and tragically unable to convey their love.

The distortion or lack of precision of the tales about their childhood is a totally understandable fact if we think that they were too little to understand and had to protect themselves somehow from patently unfavorable conditions.

For me, understanding the Drivers of one's parents and the fragility of one's mother is a way to stop thinking that one is the outcome of some horror or of an original sin, a way to dispel a nightmare still active in one's mind.

As we have seen, almost always behind and before repeated destructive educational behaviors there is a loving intent overwhelmed by unimaginable (for a child) inabilities and muted tragedies. To discover that one has inside themselves good "seeds" is always a great relief for all and leads to a greater identification with the good part inside oneself and one's parents.

Luckily today we can see stories, tales and movies for children where the parents, even if they don't have totally acceptable behaviors, are described with a little more understanding and a wider view of their conditions. I am thinking for example of the movie *The Brave* (by Mark Andrews and Brenda Chapman, 2012) where the tragedy of mother's rejection of her tomboy daughter and the ensuing rebellion becomes a pathway to awareness and evolution for both, with an ending where the diversity of the daughter and the preoccupation of the mother are both respected.

When the parents are unable to accept their children unconditionally as they are, to respect them as individuals, they inevitably convey subtle or "double-sided" negative messages.

Usually against the qualities that they did not acquire and are therefore unconsciously opposed.

They have never liked persons with those features and therefore when a child manifests them naturally, often in a reckless way, they oppose them thinking they are doing "good" and are educating their children.

The problem is that even when the messages relate only to specific behaviors but are repeated, the parents end up throwing away the child with the dirty water, devaluating the underlying drive that the child is developing.

It is true that children often exaggerate and dramatize, but one thing is to contain and another is to disparage, one thing is to provide limits and another to crush the natural drive that is starting to express itself.

But often it's also only the behavioral examples that interfere with the development of propensities. I am thinking of the great impact on the development of the personality of children of some peculiar features of their parents, such as having a solitary and detached character or working in mortifying and too heavy conditions, or even holding too rigorous and constraining religious or political beliefs.

I also think of how some events can radically change a person's relational setup and attachment, as for example great tragedies or frequent moves from one place to another.

Other relevant factors are a family's financial situation and number of children, living in isolated areas or in a tight community, whether one lives in a stimulating environment, whether one's family is united and relations are warm and intimate, and so forth.

All these objective elements inevitably mix with the messages sent by the parents and will eventually shape the narrative that a child makes of themselves and the world, giving rise to an ever partial and unrealistic Script given the age at which it is established.

## Bibliography

Alberini C., Travaglia A. (2017) Infantile amnesia: A critical period of learning to learn and remember. In *The Journal of Neuroscience*, Jun 14; 37(24): 5783–5795.

Ammaniti M., Gallese V. (2014) *The Birth of Intersubjectivity. Psychodynamic, Neurobiology, and Self*. New York, W. W. Norton & Co.

Diamond J. (2012) *The World until Yesterday: What Can We Learn from Traditional Societies?* London, Penguin Books.

Marinopulos S. (2005) *Dans l'intime des mères* (*In the innermost of mothers*). Paris, Fayard.

Winnicott D. W. (1987) *Babies and Their Mothers*. New York, Da Capo Press.

# Chapter 8

# Group psychotherapy

While I was reading and browsing books in my library in preparation of a presentation to a congress I found these lines that I had underlined in the 1980s (40 years ago) in the book entitled *Il coraggio di Venere – The courage of Venus*, by Luigi (aka Gino) Pagliarani, a master for my generation who died in 2001:

> It leads us to reflect on what is primary. And I think that coming to the world is already a suggestion of beauty. It is Eros being born.
>
> Secondarily, and since there has been an imprinting of the recognition of original beauty, comes the experience of our flaws, the origin of ambivalence, I am beautiful and/or I am ugly. ... On this aspect psychoanalysis insisted, even the less pessimistic one.
>
> (Balint talks of a fundamental flaw, not of fundamental beauty). (1985, p. 256)

I am moved by these words, I think how I came upon them after so many years, how I underlined them then, how they have affected me without realizing it and how I can use them today with gratitude.

I think of Gino's joy of living, his ability to buck the trend, to be a jolly and optimistic psychoanalyst, but also critical and aggressive, I think of how fruitful his role in groups was, of his generosity. Of how he stimulated me to become what I am today.

I think that to include this quotation here is the best way to honor a father and to open a chapter where I will try to explain why for me psychotherapy is better done in a group, except for some cases that I will discuss later.

After over 30 years spent working with this methodology, my colleagues, all Transactional Analysts, and I at the Centro Berne in Milan have no doubts left on the efficacy of group therapy and on this agree also the patients that left us more than satisfied, even those who had initially tried individual psychotherapy at our center or elsewhere.

The need for a group derives from the premises of this book, in the sense that in the relations that sooner or later inevitably develop in a group, patients can experiment with new relational experiences that start with repairing the

DOI: 10.4324/9781003303831-8

relations that had frustrated their natural propensities and later favor the construction of new modes of relating.

A group, especially when one starts meeting it, is an environment where one can find sympathy for one's distress, difficulties and distorted and invalidating Script adaptations but also, at a deeper level, is the place where one can at last find acceptance for one's original natural self that emerges, with difficulty but inevitably, open, available, trusting, and ready to make new experiences.

The group progressively becomes a laboratory where one can contact one's relational problems, the ones that are known and the ones that need to be discovered and in the end the group becomes the training grounds where one can experiment with new behaviors.

The original beauty mentioned by Pagliarani can at last emerge, be welcome, celebrated and consolidated by the group with the joy and satisfaction that it would have deserved from the very start.

But let us make one step at a time.

For me a therapeutic course is a journey of rebirth and rediscovery of natural relational happiness, a pathway of joy and surprise, like reopening the forgotten rooms of one's innocence.

Human beings are obviously not responsible for their limitations; their only responsibility, I think it was St. Augustine who said it, lies in not doing, it is abstention, isolation, individualism but in this case, we should also always ask how is it possible that what in nature is enthusiasm, group spirit, liveliness, declines during growth and becomes passivity and retreat.

An ever-present goal of my work is to recover the original drives and the relevant relational capabilities.

I try to help my patients recover a good psychic functioning but always inside a relation that reactivates both the natural "friendship" toward fellow persons and the wish to live one's life fully. This is why we work in a group; because *the medium is the message*, and the message we give to patients with group therapy is that without the capacity to establish positive relations, there is no growth: individual awareness or increased self-esteem are not enough.

To live *is* to learn to be happy in a world inhabited by other persons where each person can find a balance between self-realization and belonging, between conservation and evolution.

The "means of transportation" we use, individual or collective, are an indication of the journey we intend to make.

Any difficulty once shared is already therapy. The open expression of one's emotions is already therapy, to reveal one's past and one's present and to find true understanding is already therapy, just like seeing that others recognize our innocence.

It is already therapy to feel with others the wellbeing of a trusting surrender, to laugh about one's limitations, to accept each other, to try to change here and now with others, to feel loving feelings toward persons like you and different from you, to be publicly praised for one's qualities, to find compassion for one's difficulties.

All this is already therapy because it is the rediscovery of the common essence of our humanity, on one side, and of the possibility to live it with others, on the other.

A therapy group is a theater where we put on stage old scripts with their memories.

Then the various memories are compared, verified, often integrated and changed; our memories are fed by the memories of others and are further stimulated to emerge from the fog of the past.

And everything happens in front of an audience interested in sharing the show that is always also partially theirs.

In a group we can highlight and understand the reasons that led us to write those stories and not others; we are free from prohibitions and shadows the old characters that we had to deny, to pass them to an author, partially or totally new, the new Self.

Each actor is no longer only a performer of a role written in the past but becomes its author.

In a group the participants share, verify, experiment a new life project in the here and now so that each actor is "trained" and ready to express it in the other groups and communities without which we could not survive.

When a person shows their intention to change or when simply facing a problem of which they do not yet understand the outline, they find seven or eight persons who listen with attention, participation, and often experience in the same difficulties.

They do not give advice but help to understand, offer their views and experiences, sympathize, and then root for them.

One feels also in the body the exceptional closeness given by physical contact and sharing pain but also the jolly camaraderie that empathizes with the joy of change.

A group applauds good news, takes and gives back energy, optimism, trust.

A group is not an ideal world; often there are conflicts and misunderstandings that need to be cleared, but is at least it is a new family that welcomes a castaway and helps them reread the past with different, smart eyes, reflecting a part that hadn't yet developed: the Adult Ego State.

The persons making group therapy slowly learn that their only "fault" is their "original beauty" that had only the daring to express itself fully in order to become a human being that for their nature cannot but wish to taste the forbidden fruit of the tree of good and evil.

It is our vitality, our curiosity, our wish to know and love, our drive to evolution that makes us leave the garden of Eden where the "master" is a God that wants us to submit. And what Eden can it be without exploration and knowledge of good and evil?

From then on, but we do it also as children; we started to hide and cover our-selves, to spy instead of looking and seeing openly. We do it to avoid "Judgment".

Why should a child blame themselves when they longed for the supreme good, what "shame" should they cover after having been rejected for their exu-berant, dangerous and unbearable vitality and beauty?

Let us think of those children trained to hate and kill or simply those trained to look at others with contempt and to think arrogantly only of themselves!

To change the image internalized in our past and to develop the potential that has never been exercised offers irrepressible joy to a person sentenced unjustly who is offered a new trial after many years.

They cry for joy when the sentence is overturned and are applauded by the audience; the judge they had unfortunately believed to be right had in turn been proved incompetent and "corrupt" for a long time.

That judge (who was a parent, a family, a culture) was in turn tired, busy, ignorant, sick, dispirited, psychically frail at the time; they too had been sen-tenced to a loveless and joyless life.

They even though the law was on their side and they were its embodiment, they were in the end just a poor sucker with a feeble mind, like many others.

Compassion for that judge is, as we will see, the last step for recovering the whole of our primary love.

Because there is no peace without having recovered that parent, Ogre or Witch, an "object" that was also, in part or totally, good and lovable.

But it is with them that we have to come to terms.

It is them we have to re-start loving at the end of therapy.

To rewrite the past concerns mostly them and their existence that quite often has been even worse than ours.

And most of all, it concerns what we have done of *ourselves* "in our fights with them" without realizing it.

Technically our therapy groups once started go on living forever, patients after a period of individual sessions enter a group and stay with it until they have ended their therapy.

This means that each patient enters a group that has been existing for years and has a relatively consolidated culture, so they find, at least in part and at various degrees, typical, well run values and behaviors that represent the best way to make group therapy (a method) but also each patient's possible objec-tives (goals): Authenticity, Intimacy, Responsibility, Respect, Trust, Sympathy.

The values of an existing group correspond to the growth goals of its members.

These goals coincide roughly with the required needs of the five character armors outlined by bioenergetics (Lowen, 1975, Marchino, 1995): the schizoid character who was denied the right of existence; the oral who lacked nourish-ment; the psychopath who needs to be supported in their identity; the masoch-ist who was denied the right of being themselves; the rigid unable to let go in loving relations.

At the beginning patients find it difficult to express themselves in this way and each kind of character will reach their limits, especially when the group is "mature".

At times they will feel out of place, or incompetent or even lost in a "madhouse" but this will become an opportunity (like all other difficulties or obstacles or frustrations one meets) to reflect on one's responses, relational life, attitudes, Script.

Since these values are necessary for good communication, sooner or later they will, however, emerge both in discussing the problems of one member in particular or reflecting on the functioning mode of the group as a whole.

In this sense for me group therapy has always a double value: on one side the "treatment" of an individual, on the other the "treatment" of group phenomena.

One of the most fundamental elements of a group is the possibility of sharing with all its members the problems and solutions of one member in the "here and now".

It does not always happen, but when one reflects on some of the themes that we will see later on, the return on group functioning is immediate also because one has the chance of seeing the desired behaviors applied immediately.

If a person needs to adopt a behavior of retreat or passivity or secretiveness or abstention from work, there is nothing wrong; we should only verify the usefulness and temporary need for it in the developmental path of that person.

The investment in terms of time, frequency, punctuality, active participation in the group made by patients is part of the therapy and therefore an element that proves their psychological condition at that time.

The group's relational climate (where at the forefront is the implementation of these values) is however an arrival point that cannot be taken for granted; it will never be fully reached and perceived as definitive also because new members will join bringing along their problems, new stimuli and old habits.

Let us now analyze these values.

## The values of the therapy group

### *Authenticity*

The capacity of showing oneself as one is, with the maximum possible aware sincerity.

We are not all aware of all aspects of our life, we often tell ourselves "stories", we defend, withdraw, hide behind our false selves, at the beginning of therapy we are so ironclad inside our definitions of ourselves, of the world and of our story that we believe are inevitable and monolithic, that it seems illusory for us to be fully authentic, which means totally natural and intimate.

All the false selves, all the Victims, Rescuers, and Persecutors (Karpman, 1968, Cosso, 2014, Magrograssi, 2014) are sincere, all the depressed really believe they are worth nothing, all the narcissists believe that they don't feel, all the paranoid believe they are living in a hostile and dangerous world.

Since they are unaware they are sincere but authenticity is something else.

At the beginning in a group we invite persons to be authentic in the sense of not hiding what they know of themselves.

Even if it is an illusory and distorted opinion, as we sometimes discover, it is however important that we play fair and do not lie voluntarily to the group.

With time the word *authenticity* takes up another deeper color, as persons engage and open up, it becomes the free expression of their selves, it becomes the simple and frank contact of their emotional life with self-awareness, it becomes a permission to show one's authentic emotions when one thinks it proper and useful for the current situation.

Authenticity is not a free expression of oneself, it is not the shamelessness of a person always showing what they feel when they feel it, but it is contact with one's emotional life and with the truthfulness of one's actions, always in a context of respect and relational sensitivity.

Authenticity means to overcome the defenses we have created to hide or change our essence of human beings, to recover the adequacy of our natural emotions to the current situation, both in terms of quality and of duration and "volume".

It means to relinquish ancient emotional responses – "parasites" – (Stewart and Joines, 1996, English, 1992) with which we had to substitute the responses that would have come natural in childhood. It means to rediscover and reactivate for what is possible our devalued propensities, accepting openly our limitations and our current condition.

Authenticity means to stop trying to be PERFECT, PLEASING, HURRIED or STRONG, prey of superhuman EFFORTS to be accepted by others and feeling and showing ourselves as OK in the way we "have been able to become".

Therapy helps to recognize and change our limits, and this is exciting, but we will always need the awareness to "have to" accept to love ourselves and others for what the story of each one has made possible.

For someone authenticity consists in giving value to their reflective shyness, not trying to become an actor on stage; for others it means to recognize their exuberance giving it a proper expression instead of feeling guilty; for others it means to discover a part of themselves that had been marginalized and give it adequate space. To let our authentic identity emerge we need always both expansion and limits, both for evolving and for preserving.

### Intimacy

The capacity to relate deeply and authentically with others, and with oneself; it is the familiarity, confidentiality, closeness of a person who feels part of humankind in its deepest sense of sharing the condition of faultiness and beauty, uncertainty and potential, impermanence and uniqueness. Intimacy is a relation without hidden claims and requests, where the offer of oneself is only an invitation to communication, more or less deep, but always shared in the moment it happens: we are intimate while being silent, making love, teaching and learning, working side by side, feeling similar emotions and sharing them, sharing suffering and winking while joking, gossiping and forming alliances. We are intimate when closeness is between persons that let themselves be seen and look with interest at what is taking place in that moment.

Intimacy is the "here and now" of persons united by the thread, that can be thin but is always strong and solemn, of our clear humanity.

Intimacy has many enemies. First of all, manipulation, the true meaning of what we call appearance, which is making others believe, willfully or not, what we are not. This is why in groups we take great care of the inconsistency between what we say and how our body moves, how we use words, the tone of voice, face mimics, all those attitudes that seem to contradict our words or let emerge what we don't know.

But we don't want to unmask, expose or worse correct language or behavior – activities that are totally against therapy because they invite persons to "control" their behaviors and therefore be less simple and authentic – but rather we want to help persons understand what they are truly expressing, let emerge the deep drive that they might be "trying" to express but somehow hamper with another part of themselves.

Inconsistencies, but we should rather say the so-called defenses, are only the conflict between healthy developmental needs and the opposed effort at staying within the confines of more usual and well-known Scripts.

Respectful and always available persons (Complying) who, for example, are always apologizing for their behavior, are not truly kind and helpful, are not truly altruistic and generous, they are simply unable to show openly their fear of being judged, are hampered in expressing their discomfort, cannot show their difference.

In this sense, their deference is a form of manipulation to make them welcome and accepted.

Enemies of intimacy are also haste, superficiality, to want all immediately, competitivity.

There are no shortcuts for a person's evolution: performing and sharp therapists or dazzling and cathartic flashes of emotion are not enough.

We need slowness to feel, depth not to be content with what is comfortable and usual, *sweetness* to walk along warmly and respectfully.

I want to stress these values – "lentius, profundius, suavius" (slower, deeper, gentler)– that Alexander Langer (1994), one of the most relevant leaders of the first European environmental movement considered indispensable for our future of peace, integration and happiness as opposed to the Olympian keywords "citius, altius, fortius." (faster, higher, stronger).

RESPONSIBILITY, that is also autonomy.

It seems odd, but it is truly rare for a person that initially comes for help to do it with a clear idea of how little we are in charge of our destiny. To feel responsible of what one does, of what one feels or thinks, is truly difficult for many persons.

But one of the final goals of psychotherapy is to feel responsible of one's life.

We have all been brought up by others, others have welcomed our "natural precursors" and have changed them into inclinations acceptable for them, others at a given age have seen us and chosen us for what we have become. It should be relevant for all to look at ourselves in the mirror and ask "Do I like it this way?"

To feel responsible means to master one's emotions and gestures, one's relations, one's more or less codified ways of thinking.

To know how to choose, leaving our familiar plans and our "basic configurations", means to become autonomous (for what is possible) from the constraints of our past; it means to eliminate from our vocabulary phrases like "you make me feel sad" or "what you say is offensive" or worse "this job, this woman, this relation, this story, this cold and cloudy weather … is killing me".

Too obvious but necessary is adding that to be superstitious or to believe in horoscopes is the total denial of our power, self-esteem and possibility/ability to determine our life and our autonomy.

### Respect

Is the condition described by the transactional slogan "I am OK, you are OK" created by Eric Berne, the founder of TA, because he wanted to take the "patient" off the couch and make them sit like a "person" in front of him in order to finally have a dialogue together on what "seems to be OK in his life".

Every once in a while, I like to sit next to the patients; it feels like walking arm in arm to indicate that we are together trying to understand what is going on and what course we should take. Respect is first of all attention to the person's diversity, values, beliefs, but also the enhancement of their resources and abilities and understanding of the difficulties they meet in their course of evolution and therapy.

Berne (1961, 1966) asserted that every person, even those with the most damaged psychic functioning, still retained sufficient reflective and rational capacities in their Adult Ego State with which to form a productive alliance.

Years of clinicians' (not only psychoanalysts') attitudes of superiority with their "arcane" knowledge jealously guarded and not understandable for most persons, with their symbols that could be understood only from their reference theory, with undisputable interpretations derived from a dogmatic wisdom, worked against psychotherapy because they devalued the competence of those asking for help – patients by definition – and mythicized the knowledge of therapists.

Respect means attention to what a person says; it is a way of listening that gives value also to the unspoken as well as to the spoken, a stimulus for reflection and protection in order to change in the direction that that person wishes and for as long they wish it.

Group therapy is a journey during which all members must learn to show what they want, where all the participants will leave the last word to each person and no one will ever say "I think that for you it would be better to …", but they will express what they consider useful by saying "For me it is better to …"

Respect from the therapist means also not to hide their knowledge both by explaining what relational and psychological competence they are using to put all group members in the condition to understand themselves and the others, and explaining what they are technically doing.

Our work makes use of various techniques, exercises, guided reflections, role play, actions aimed at making explicit, remembering, regressing, and all of them have a meaning and a goal that group members need to understand and share in order to want to use them properly with their modes and rhythms.

The same applies to what some psychotherapies call resistances: to respect persons means also to accept their difficulties, to get rid once and for all of this blaming attitude that calls unfit for analysis or hostile or counter-dependent or in a negative transference or resistant whoever simply finds it hard to follow the therapist's demands.

Each person relies, cooperates, rationalizes, learns and shows themselves or retreats, struggles, doesn't understand and even forgets what they said depending on their possibilities.

Respect means also not to judge persons from their willingness to follow and listen to their guru with dedication and humility or even creatively and actively.

Patients ask for help often because they do not how to trust, don't know how to believe in themselves and not even in their therapist, they ask for help because they are passive, counter-dependent, hostile, "off-putting" or even "ugly, dirty, and nasty".

If they struggle, and it is normal if they do, we cannot say that they are unfit for therapy and leave them to their destiny or even think that this is not the right moment to start.

We have to keep our hand extended with patience and acceptance, there to be taken.

Sooner or later it will happen but it will be all the more possible if we will respect their difficulties.

At times therapists run too fast, cannot find the right distance or the right rhythm, they want to feel successful and therefore they demand that everything happens according to their expectations. In the end, they are not accepting the persons as they are.

## Trust

This is probably one of the most widely varying values in groups, but also in individual therapies. It tends to follow the successes and difficulties in changing.

If a person comes to therapy, it should mean that they have seen at least a faint opportunity to tackle their distress and therefore they have at least in part believed in our possibilities.

At times we need to leverage on this little element to stimulate trust in ourselves and in them.

There are personalities that revel in devaluing treatment and therapists, in particular those who at the beginning rely on our reputation as magical healers.

Sooner or later disappointment will take the form of a powerful weapon that will try to bring us down as we fly so high, they think, like an inflated balloon.

But we have to be steadfast, my experience and my belief in human nature help me to believe in and trust the possibilities of all persons.

At the beginning of psychotherapy, we have to openly state how things work but usually this is not enough: high expectations and haste are difficult to eradicate, as well as the subtle skepticism or the most blatant competitive challenges that are the expression of the obvious difficulty in changing one's behavior. We have to expect that; it's the Scripts, that's all.

We can do it together if we try hard enough (but what s enough?), if we listen to the flicker that Is active in our minds and hearts, if we look at how we came to this, distressed survivors.

A capable therapist always sees (and shows) under each ragged, dirty, lowly or armored disguise that original beauty that is so moving when you start seeing it and slowly recovers its shine.

And here a group is even more useful. A therapist sides with the patient but when the other members rejoice and respond positively, congratulate them for the goal reached or even recall the changes occurred when all seemed difficult, even the most self-devaluing and dejected person opens a crack in their losing Script to exclaim "Is it true? Have I changed?"

For building and maintaining trust in a group, whenever possible we should make coincide the exit of a person at the end of their therapy with the entrance of another person beginning their therapy.

The last sessions in a group are always a celebration. I always ask the person to retrace their journey, to highlight the old problems, what parts of their personality were in need of repair, what has been done and what has proved truly helpful.

A further way for crystallizing change and an opportunity for me to give feedback to the person along with some reinforcing memory.

The person leaving thanks the other members and the therapist; some write a letter, others give a personalized and meaningful gift, we always hug and are moved.

The closing of a therapy that has lasted for years with persons with whom one shared joy and pain once a week is an epic and memorable moment.

The new members are surprised, most of them do not expect it.

Even if I always explain beforehand the functioning of a group, it is barely possible to convey the happiness of these moments, the joy mixed with the sadness of parting and the fear for the loss of such a deep and now customary support, that is rare and difficult to build "out there".

But most of all they don't expect the quality of the recognitions that persons exchange and the relational climate that makes the goals reached concretely perceivable albeit in varying degrees.

The new members are usually surprised and envious of what they see, while the old members that are leaving look at them with compassion, but that joy and those hugs are always a general nourishment (for the therapist too, obviously) that helps to look with trust and optimism at the journey one is starting.

### Sympathy/solidarity

It is almost funny to see people surprised when they learn that we make group therapy. If they have never experienced anything of that kind and I ask them if they are willing, if they agree with the dates I suggest, if they want to start thinking about it, they look at me with great skepticism and a certain suspicion: "Will it help me?" "Am I fit for it?" "And why should I?"

There are persons that accept it directly and already know that we almost always suggest group therapy, but most of them are negatively surprised and ask questions mostly about the other participants.

Usually what they simply don't see is the most relevant dimension of group work: the opportunity to find acceptance, support and hence sympathy and help to face one's problems. In general they ask "But who cares about my problems" – on the depressive side – or "But why should I have to listen to others explaining their problems; is it going to be boring?" – on the narcissistic/paranoid side.

This low consideration of relational possibilities tells a lot about the marginalization imposed to human suffering by our society.

Distress, pain, disability, diseases in general or mental illness, but even at a lower level the difficulties posed by daily life are experienced and treated like a private matter that needs to be hidden, of which one is ashamed. To talk about it in public seems quite difficult and almost useless.

Usually it takes months before I suggest to a person to join a group; in fact I need to have established a solid trusting relationship that is already good enough to allow them to make this decision without too much prejudice and without creating too much detachment in the relation.

We will later return to the questions posed by entering a group; here I only want to add that sympathy is the biggest positive surprise for all. For the sociological reasons I was describing above, persons don't expect such a positive and welcoming encounter with the others, nor that participation and brotherliness can be achieved easily and turn out warm and authentic.

When a new person enters a group the others introduce themselves first and in addition to their relevant personal information, I ask them to tell also what brought them to therapy, what they wanted to change and how they are doing at the moment.

This highlights immediately the similarities between participants, what they have in common and shows to the newcomer how each member makes their problems explicit.

Persons don't expect that a surgeon can be afraid of operating or that a teacher can struggle with their aggressive tendency or that a mother of three can feel anxious because she sacrificed her life for her children or that a successful manager can lead a loveless life or that an actor cannot express their emotions or a businessman after years of success can feel they have no goal in life.

Now that I think of it, what would persons sound like if I described them by their pathologies?

I was talking of a phobic obsessive, a paranoid, a depressed, a narcissist, an alexithymic, a manic depressive. Those who do not know group therapy think they will meet aliens, more or less imagined or described as I did above, certainly not persons just like them. They imagine disturbed persons as they saw them in the movies or as they think they could find them in psychiatry handbooks, but don't expect the actual distress of actual persons, alive and filled with extraordinary resources.

On the other hand, we are almost all like them, like when we pick a fight with someone while driving just because the other driver is an anonymous stranger and we can despise them for their behavior but if we get nearer, at a closer look, we are all the same: in a hurry, nervous and we find it really difficult to thaw the ice screen that separates us.

But the miracles of brotherhood do happen.

When the distance becomes shorter and the ice melts, persons in the deep of their being show what they "potentially" are: sympathetic, intimate, cooperating.

Under a storm or near a hospital bed we end up being close and ready to hold hands.

And this is a beautiful discovery, fast for some and relatively slow and difficult for others, but it is always the happy and satisfying outcome of group work.

So when one cries, there is always someone, in addition to the therapist obviously, ready to hug and comfort; when someone is angry there is another who can understand even when disagreeing; when one is scared there is always someone who felt the same emotion and confirms that one can get free from fear just like they did.

The group can become the closeness that had always been lacking, the place where unconditional acceptance from other humans, in addition to stimulating the emergence of our potential it allows also criticism, disapproval, open confrontations that do not become a destructive and competitive fight.

But group psychotherapy is also the discovery of how community is lacking in our everyday lives, how we need others and how belonging is a crucial drive that it is difficult to forgo without suffering. It also shows how much joy of life we are missing out if we are unable to build relations of sympathy, comfort, and sharing in "real life".

Group psychotherapeutic work in the end becomes also a political message: there is no progress, no evolution without cooperation, equality and brotherhood.

Let us not forget where we are in the evolutionary story of our species: "liberté, egalité, fraternité". Where freedom is also freedom from the constraints of the past.

But what does a therapist do in a group? Below I'll try to give a schematic description of their work to give at least an idea although I know that such a list cannot exhaust the subject.

## The activities of a group therapist

### Toward patients

Creates an alliance already in the individual phases preceding the entrance in the group.

Draws up a contract, defines a first general goal of therapy.

Listens to the background noise, the group's climate, understands its phases and needs.

Observes what happens in the "here and now" in order to understand how the persons are acting in the group.

Looks at individual gestures, positions, expressions to understand problems, also the ones not yet expressed.

Uses what happens in the "here and now" to improve self-awareness.

Favors direct, expressive, authentic communication.

Uses therapeutic techniques and methods in order to favor:

- The creation of a group structure
- Socialization and mutual acceptance
- Recognitions and feedback among members, favoring the communication and free expression of emotions
- Self-awareness and responsibility for one's actions and experiences
- The ability for proprioceptive introspection, distinguishing between thoughts, emotions, sensations and fantasies
- The ability to understand others and to be empathic
- Authenticity
- Learning new desirable behaviors

- Creativity and self-confidence
- Flexibility, that is the ability to be Adult, Parent, Child, depending on the situation and on one's needs and the needs of others

### Toward the group

The therapist favors, first of all with their behavior, a relational world characterized by the values I consider crucial: Authenticity, Intimacy, Responsibility, Respect, Trust, and Sympathy.

Stimulates listening, unconditional acceptance of each person and their mistakes and difficulties (I am OK, you are OK), awareness and "unashamed" knowledge of oneself, the wish to evolve and learn.

In this sense, but taking care of not putting themselves in a negative light and therefore lose authoritativeness, recognizes their own mistakes and difficulties, also disclosing, if appropriate, events of their past (if they stimulated growth) and elements of their lives.

This too is a way to make the hindrances and bothers of life acceptable because they happened and happen to the therapist too.

There is no reason but narcissism to show oneself as omnipotent and faultless, while instead being relatively open and genuine invites just as much transparency, spontaneity, and acceptance of oneself.

Authenticity and intimacy are values that a therapist promotes also with their habitual attitudes, obviously without ostentation and complacency.

They should not let themselves be seen different from what they are: an impassible, mysterious and faraway myth that cannot be engaged and stimulated, that does not show their emotions, does not show their feelings with measure and simplicity.

To be moved, to have fun, to worry and to rejoice, to be outraged and sympathetic, even to admit to have been wrong and change one's mind is always very useful to build group culture.

With the great unpassable limit, each action by the therapist must be "necessary" and "useful" for the persons and at the same time must express a positive universality totally consistent with the values that we want to convey. A therapist also facilitates closeness and adult attachment modes among the patients and between the patients and themselves. Helps them experiment and lets positive and negative transferences emerge, helps them to read their historical motivations and overcome repetition.

Progressively develops a new positive Parent in the group that will at first be represented by the therapist and by the rules set and in time by the shared culture that will be created through consolidated practices that are explicitly discussed and approved.

Lastly, favors with their exemplary behavior characterized by Power (assertiveness, authoritativeness, consistency), Permission (let do, accept, exhort) and Protection (care, defense, support) the spontaneous exchanges of recognition and physical and verbal stroking, contributions and feedback, also critical, provided they have a positive intention, and the manifestation of emotions, the expression of requests and needs, rejections, denials or conflicts.

In this way in the group one learns to relate, to understand deeply and to accept with "sympathy" the Other as a human being.

## Ten reasons to make group therapy

1. A group is a realistic theater where each person can show the relational modes they use also outside it. This highlights the attitudes that in individual therapy are mostly put into words and often not highly considered. At the same time we let emerge the transferences with familiar figures, not only parents.
2. It stimulates positive feedback and recognitions from different persons, at times the other group members are listened to and accepted more than the therapist, whose positive contributions are often taken for granted.
3. It develops wellbeing, attachment, positivity, freeing endorphins when members share values, thoughts, and emotions. It gives value to becoming a fellow human being and getting close to the others.
4. It provides a miniature social universe, a new family, where one can enact new and varied relational modes, triggers parenting toward persons in difficulty, the wish to spend time together, rationality and discussion of one's opinions, ascertaining limitations and defaults in one's personality.
5. It favors contacts and the expression of regressive and deep parts of oneself deriving from stimuli or questions from others, it helps to overcome shame and guilt, it relieves from isolation.
6. It makes it possible to use different techniques (psychodrama, Gestalt, bioenergetics, group dream analysis, role play, etc.) where the presence of other persons is necessary.
7. It shows the need for harmony between focusing on oneself (self-realization) and attention to others (belonging). It allows to experiment different proper distances, intimacy and solitary reflection.
8. It highlights the existential issues common to humans by comparing different views and positions on themes such as life and death, injustice, illness, distress, the meaning of life and so on.
9. It unites and joins in distress, making one's unease explicit and allowing to escape one's shameful privateness to find closeness and belonging. The group accepts fragility as a human condition, does not consider it weakness but helps to accept one's finitude and fragility.
10. It stimulates mutual feedback among members (in addition to those provided by the therapist) on one's self-image and thus widens and deepens, integrates and at times contradicts the view that each member has of themselves, thus contributing to the knowledge of one's identity.

I put at the end of this list what I consider one of the most important elements of group therapy: the opportunity to expand the information that each member receives.

Patients, in fact, are a very powerful resource available to all to check one's image of oneself that is often quite distorted and univocal.

And it is a decisive opportunity, in particular in an advanced phase of therapy to stimulate a new "narrative" of oneself overcoming the script rigidities that built up in years.

It is a common experience in therapeutic groups that the propensity to change is activated even only by listening to and watching the others, discovering common drives and desires within oneself (the Natural Child Ego State) but also very personal automatic actions that derive from the progressive learning that in time crystallized and settled forming important parts of personality (Adapted, Adequate, Subject or Rebellious Child, Normative and Affective Parent, positive and negative, and Adult). In this sense we can consider therapy as an activity aimed at affecting the structural contents of personality and behavioral functioning.

## Structural contents

Structural contents learned in childhood form a set of emotional experiences, relevant events, usually unconscious decisions and opinions on oneself, the others and the world, information settled in neuronal circuits connected among them in the early phases of life.

When frustrations are prolonged or especially radical, it is clear that natural propensities can be more or less inhibited and deviated toward substitute areas and defensive behaviors.

All this is justified and rationalized with biased values and opinions that reinforce learning.

For a child fixations, traumas, confusion, abandonments, prohibitions, and conflicts become an indisputable reality, an unconscious history that settles and is confirmed in time.

Normally persons do not keep account of this deep structure, even if they act based on its assumptions.

An unsafe base, for example, makes it difficult to realize the drive to autonomy or even a real and deep love life, but at first sight we see only shyness, reluctance, a certain inwardness, and so on and even some therapists will tend to act at this first evident level.

We can develop a good awareness, help to think differently, offer alternatives, suggest small steps, but obviously if we don't change the deep fear of the primary disappointment (the prerequisite) and don't develop a new safe base, our efforts will be superficial with temporary and forced outcomes.

From the point of view of Ego States this means to check what remains of the wish to live of the Natural Child, for example.

How and how much an excessive or violent adaptation has mortified, depressed, and *subjugated* the natural propensity to love, self-determination, and so forth. Or how and how much the parents' aggressive and destructive behaviors have elicited a hostile and manic image of oneself and the world with automatic antagonistic or *rebellious* responses.

We know very well that many difficulties derive from the fact that persons are ego-syntonic with their issues and therefore often don't even perceive their limitations and end up feeling they have always been lonely rather than rejected, inadequate or wrong rather than devalued.

When the disavowal of one's nature happens very early in life and takes root, this can be highlighted and brought to attention only through regressive work to let emerge what persons do not know of themselves.

These events cannot be told nor defined because they often happened before a person had cognitive memory, before they were aware of them, even before they were able to find some alternative way to face them, before they could understand the injustice or inaccuracy of the messages received and therefore before being able to reject them.

That Adapted Child must then be "deconfused" from what they were at the origin, from what they became and what they could have become and then must slowly be accompanied to realize that buried under old acquisitions there is another Child that may have stopped suffering but is neither healthy nor happy.

The early "deviations" from healthy development of the Child part are always accompanied and supported by a strong lack of the Adult part of personality.

Fears, distorted opinions on oneself and the world and the related waivers are taken for granted so that the residual rationality can only justify them.

A child receiving a rejection of their expressions of love or exploration endeavors or assertiveness will not be able to bear the ensuing frustrations for a long time.

Sooner or later they will adapt, and their surrender will be aimed at no longer feeling the distress that always accompanies the devaluation of a natural propensity.

Other mental spaces are the outcome of meeting their caregivers' parenting and of learning their ways. In TA we include these Ego States in the term Parent, that part that children assimilate mainly by imitation and will apply to themselves and to their relations with others.

Acceptance, protection, normativity, rules for living and most of all a more or less warm attitude will be their way of taking care of themselves and others, will become that part of their personality oriented to realizing both the survival and the belonging drive with specific attention to conservation, closeness, understanding, compassion, protection, care of oneself and one's community.

It is not only the Freudian Super-Ego but something more comprehensive, not only a limit or prohibition of the child's omnipotent and narcissistic expressions, but rather a recovered balance of the limitations and Permissions required for growth.

We are born children, we become adults and in time we also learn how to be parents of ourselves and our fellow humans.

So our Parent Ego State develops also positively by learning the ability to guide us and give us realistic limits with values that are adequate to the life we want to live, with attention to our health and that of the planet, with trust in our own potential and in that of others, with the awareness of our responsibility toward our individual and collective life.

Important contributions on these issues were made by Gregoire (2007) in *Les orientament rècentes de l'Analy Transactionelle* (Recent trends in Transactional Analysis), and by Allemandri, Baldacci, Ciurli, Poidomani, Procacci and Salnitro (2012) in *Bisogni spezzati, bisogni ritrovati: Nuovi orizzonti di analisi transazionale elaborati nella bottega* di Carlo Moiso (Broken needs: Rediscovered needs).

Persons asking for help often have had internal parental patterns that were absent or helpless without knowing it, so they feel at the mercy of others, are unable to trust themselves because their parents did not trust them, they don't know how to protect themselves because they have not been protected.

Often they are unable to or do not want to have children because they don't have in themselves the sense of the developmental potential of humankind for not having been happy children.

All these contents cannot be left unchanged by therapy, we must attend to how persons take for granted the fact that the messages received have been adequate and corresponding to their nature.

To be unable to protect oneself (the Parent) is as dangerous for the human mind as is the decline in the wish to live (the Child).

Therapeutic work on the knowledge of one's historically settled contents, the comparison with what we have become and what we could have been, is all the more indispensable, the earlier we received the messages that distorted our nature.

This is in general also one of the heaviest sorrows that one sooner or later will have to feel in therapy: to learn that our parents have extended to us a sentence to unhappiness and "madness" that we have repeated and confirmed.

It is from them, in fact, that we have learned detachment, distrust, lack of care, irrationality or aggressivity.

The messages of a Parent that is mercilessly called Ogre or Witch remains steady and working inside ourselves reminding us all the time how we should be.

So our Child part, terrorized or weak, passive or angry, solitary or narcissistic, insecure or bullying, not only keeps behaving in the way it grew up but is constantly reinforced by the beliefs that probably were held by their family and that now are repeated inside them by the Parent Ego State with their recorded voices that are more or less consciously amplified: "the world is a mess", "you can no longer trust anybody", "you must be Strong, Perfect, Hurry, Please, Try hard, etc.", "you'll never make it", "control all and control yourself".

Almost all the therapeutic interventions described in this book go in this "structural" direction, not because they are the only ones, as we will see later since the main theme of this book is the treatment of love and affection, but rather because they are the ones that act more deeply on the early inhibition of love.

I want to remind readers that persons today feel great distress that is however much less serious than the one felt by a child hampered in growth who tried to avoid themselves by adapting their behaviors to the messages they received.

When persons go back to the origins of damage, they feel the old pain of the primary wounds and their tragedy appears in all its truth and severity, their crying is then exactly the cry of a child that can finally feel the distance between their natural drives and the frustrations suffered.

In these cases the group is the "new world" that welcomes, understands, sympathizes, comes very close so it can physically hug the child part of the person that now needs to feel that this pain is sacred and right, that they were not wrong when they felt destroyed by the lack of acceptance but on the contrary that what they have done to avoid those rejections was inevitable, was the proof of how their wish to survive was stronger than any abuse, violence, lack of care.

The discovery of what one could not develop of their essence as humans becomes from then on the crucial goal of one's evolution.

## Changes in behavior

As can be easily imagined, changes in behavior are almost always the first request persons make. The pain they perceive is the present one or the one accumulated for years. "I feel lonely, I can't sleep at night, I'm anxious, I lost my job, I have premature ejaculation, I have nightmares, I can't get up in the morning", are some typical complaints.

I think we should always pay attention to what is important in that moment for that person. Even when we can easily imagine and diagnose more serious problems and the underlying complexes, we should first provide an answer to the pain they are suffering "here and now".

We can build a relation of trust and progressive opening only if we deserve that trust.

I always ask myself if what I do is already a form of help: active listening, being available and welcoming, unconditional acceptance, non-judgmental, and sympathetic, often is already in itself a form of help. But it is also true that often patients want immediate and concrete changes. A good starting point is often to help them give a clear and understandable name to their difficulties.

To understand what is going on and why and, most of all, to learn to guide one's behavior feeling responsible for it gives a sense of mastery and agency that can shed light on new possibilities for change and give a new hope for happiness.

TA was born initially for this kind of interventions and the terms used to describe personality (Parent, Adult and Child with their functional qualifications Adapted, Adequate, Subject, Rebellious Child and Affective and Normative Parent, positive and negative) and the relations among persons (positive and negative Transactions, Recognitions, Games and Blackmailing System, etc.) when we explain them always become a surprising discovery that is extremely activating.

Mastering a relatively simple psychological language, that is however quite efficient, makes the patient an active participant in the process they are starting.

They feel valued for their resources and progressively capable of intervening in their changes, even if only with small steps.

To develop the ability to reflect on oneself and one's behavior, to analyze one's attitudes, to plan one's actions, to have social control of one's actions, to discover new behavioral options is what we mean by development of an Adult Ego State.

Work oriented in this direction tends to return to persons their control on themselves and their actions but also to make them aware of their more or less limiting mental habits and behavioral patterns (their Script).

In a similar way, we can intervene to highlight inhibited drives and unmet needs, and what creates fear or anxiety or depresses their Child parts.

In this case one needs to give value to suffering and distress because persons always need to be taken seriously, even more so when their emotional responses are shameful or unspeakable.

In order to have an effect and to trigger new behaviors, therapy must always understand what led to distress and change the old behaviors that induce it. We must never, except in case of danger for the person or for others, downplay the pain, consider it lighter than it is or, worse, sweeten it; our primary task is to give a voice to the wounded child and together with them try to reconstruct the story of their suffering, first of all the present one and, if proper, the ancient, structural, deep, archaic one.

Lastly, but this is just a brief mention of what should be done "here and now" at the behavioral level, we can address the Parental parts, understanding what parts are useful and healthy.

As we know, we learn to take care of ourselves from the many figures of authority we have met, first of all our parents.

As children we have all played mummy and daddy, we have learned care, affection and even ethics and socialization and how to be exacting, or yielding, tolerant or intolerant with ourselves and others.

When facing a present problem, it is always surprising to see how we are parents of ourselves and how we force on ourselves some behaviors rather than others.

It is often incredible how with age we tend to repeat the modes of our parents, even when we have been quite in contrast with them when we were young.

A reflection on these aspects has the same effect of work on the Child part; it truly recovers the chance of becoming masters of ourselves, to reflect and ask, "But am I still in agreement with the way I grew up?"

I stop here because I don't want to write a handbook, but I want to stress before closing this chapter that, beyond obvious simplifications, when we talk of Ego States we are talking of rather arbitrary clusters of states of the mind that are given colloquial names but still are universal functions of personality; we are talking of areas of the mind that neurophysiology is currently trying to locate in our brain.

What we need to do is optimize the Adult part that, aware of what takes place in the here and now, knowing how to listen to and understand the Child's natural drives, clears them from the useless prohibitions (Injunctions) learned in childhood, and enacts them in the realistic conditions of its present (Goulding and Goulding, 1976, 1979).

And we need also to build a system of rules and prohibitions that is adequate to one's characteristics and at the same time in harmony with the world around.

If, after having understood this, one cannot change, then it will be necessary to start a longer and deeper structural therapeutic work that might prove painful but also exciting and triumphant, like finding a pearl in a shell in the deep of the sea under a layer of mud and detritus.

### Some limitations of group therapy

I have often wondered what is the other side of the coin.

In my years of practice, it has happened to me to feel dissatisfied with what I was doing and somehow I felt the impulse to do something more or something different.

I realized that this happened especially when I had the feeling that a group remained at a superficial level.

We know very well that it is possible that a person hides inside a group, doesn't talk much and is reserved and often a confrontation on these issues can prove neither useful nor effective.

Many persons need pauses; they need to let change settle in, they need rest, and this depends mostly on the situation and on their Script, but I must confess that I noticed that often in groups we risk dwelling a little too much on the essential and neglecting details that in an individual therapy would be given more time to be explored (at least in theory).

Sometimes in groups persons tend to concentrate their interventions on some issues that are more popular or urgent rather than on other themes.

This isn't in itself a negative aspect but the suspicion that individual therapy could provide more space to introspection than group therapy still remains in me like a parasite thought.

There are various ways to limit these risks and the following are the ones I use most often.

If I feel that a person in the group needs to enter more in themselves and listen to their deeper and subtler emotional reactions, I protect them, inviting them to give themselves permission to dwell in the uncertainty, to take their time and I invite also the others to do the same.

I also ask the others if they agree in leaving more space to someone that is working less, so I stress the need for silence, for being inside oneself, for feeling better, for letting one's mind wonder among feelings and sensations.

For many persons to learn to feel and think, even without a specific intention to action or to an immediate and concrete result, is a great permission: "you can be important", "you can feel", "you can take your time".

As I must have said many times before, therapy must not be only reporting or telling but is most of all happening "here and now" that is activated, felt, and expressed.

Then there is always the possibility of adding also some individual sessions between group meetings; for some persons this means to have some exclusivity in the relation and to feel they have a link with the therapist, but individual sessions can also be necessary to "let go" in a more protected situation and dare penetrate unknown internal worlds that are felt as dangerous.

In any case, it is only the therapist that can decide whether they are necessary depending on each person's course.

Sometimes I accept a request because I understand that it can be a developmental step, a permission they give themselves to ask for recognition and specific attention; in other cases I discuss it with the group or on the phone to see if it wouldn't instead be better to talk about it in the group even if it is difficult. This too can be a developmental step if it means to give oneself permission of being intimate, trust the others, even facing something that one considered impossible to say and very private.

After individual sessions, however, the patient always reports the reasons of this choice to the group.

The depth of our work, that for me means to have a chance to access the oldest experiences and feelings and to express freely the deepest genuine emotions, should always be considered a goal to be reached for persons and groups, not a given.

We need to accept to spend some time in rituals and entertainment (light banter, recipes, sports and shows and more) in order to get there. Sooner or later we can decide to notice this and analyze it if it becomes a flight from therapeutic work but always with caution and measure.

If our goal for groups is to build and maintain a culture that favors trust, authenticity, and depth, each member must have their specific course protected, accepted and carried out with care.

## We are a wonder of dormant opportunities

Stanislas Dehaene, one of the most brilliant contemporary scientists, teacher of experimental cognitive psychology at the Collège de France, wrote in 2014:

> The discovery that a word or a digit can travel throughout the brain, bias our decisions, and affect our language networks, all the while remaining unseen, was an eye-opener for many cognitive scientists. We had underestimated the power of the unconscious.
>
> (p. 74)

Better late than never, I would comment.

> The outcome of all these experiments is clear: our brain hosts a set of clever unconscious devices that constantly monitor the world around us and assign it values that guide our attention and shape our thinking. ... Only the most relevant events draw our attention and gain a chance to enter our consciousness. Below the level of our awareness, our unconscious brain ceaselessly evaluates dormant opportunities, testifying that our attention largely operates in a subliminal manner.
>
> (p. 79)

What we call Ego States are then as many as the possible aggregations of meaning, tightly connected to one another in our mind, that happened in the past and are happening in the present.

They are all present at the same time, conscious and unconscious, which for our therapeutic practice means immediately or hardly accessible to our Adult consciousness.

The scientific discovery of the unconscious dimension of our mind and at the same time of our ability to aggregate experiences and to activate ourselves without being aware that this can be both positive and negative, appropriate to the event or not, highlights some of the most striking psychoanalytical intuitions.

It explains and confirms how difficult it is to make a real deep change without reaching the awareness of what unconsciously affected and affects our experience and change its assumption, all the more so when this touches on crucial aspects of our humanity such as drives and functions of personality.

I really like the concept of dormant opportunities; Ego States are numerous and are both early limiting decisions that oriented us toward unconscious neurotic solutions but also, and this is what I want to stress in this book, healthy drives that need to be reactivated.

In other words, in our ebullient or sedated unconscious there are still curious, loving, assertive, willful, rightly angry or disappointed, sad or scared Ego States that can be brought back to the surface to understand what we are lacking.

Our rational part and our very limited conscious attention quite often do not know this until through emotional or bodily experiences we manage to reactivate those information circuits that going deeper in our upside-down funnel we throw light on the wide sea of our past vitality, primary loves and dormant propensities.

That universal self, so large, powerful and full of unexpressed potential that always survives hidden inside ourselves is a leafy wood full of nice surprises.

We do not look for monsters inside ourselves, we go and free the species Self, the nascent beauty of Eros.

At times, if a person is desperately crying, the therapist's hug will be enough to reopen a bodily contact that had been frozen for years and to reactivate genuine emotions or healthy behaviors; at other times we will need a more continuous and delicate work; at others it will be a sudden flash, a mysterious insight triggered by an event in the group; at others it will be a movie that triggers the nostalgia for a happy past.

To recognize unconscious Ego States, to understand their rationale, their past need and current influence on life to try and change them to improve our lives is the goal of psychotherapy.

It is a process that can be never-ending since innumerable are the possible neuronal aggregates that settled and are active in our mental life as well as the revolutions we meet in the course of our life.

The tip of the iceberg is only what reaches awareness, voluntary attention and, if it's not just a drop in the ocean, it is certainly a small fraction of what lurks beneath: 16 billion cortical neurons.

A therapy group certainly cannot change an economic system that sentences persons to the paroxysm of performance, initiative, action in a total inability to be themselves (these are the drivers I described above: BE STRONG, HURRY, BE PERFECT, PLEASE, TRY HARD), but it can favor the awareness that all this is inhuman, meaningless, and very far from what can make a human being happy and realized and maybe it can help us to make different choices, non-conformist, political but also healthy and existential.

There is also a phenomenon that always happens when persons are part of a therapy group, an inevitable and enormous change in their way of looking at others that is related with perception. When we meet someone at the beginning we can have a very negative impression, we see a behavior and judge it on the basis of our preferences or idiosyncrasies.

Very often we don't like the persons that represent parts of ourselves that we have denied, those who can afford attitudes that are prohibited to us, in a word our shadow or those who represent values far from ours or persons with evident relational problems or of whom we are afraid. We are all human beings; sensitive and affectable and very often with the habit of giving value to ourselves because we are different from the others.

But then it always happens that, as that person in therapy unveils their deepest problems, as we learn the story of their existence, as we discover and understand why they are different and peculiar, once our armor is removed, ice melts, defenses are lowered, grandiosity is left aside by the conceited ones, and the humble ones stop trying to make themselves accepted, we end up inevitably finding that those human beings are ... just like ourselves.

Like ourselves also in the parts that we gave up while growing up.

We see the True Self of a Natural Child so close to our way of living that we feel they are our siblings.

And this always happens to those who join a group, and they are always surprised in varying degrees at so much humanity. Many persons have never been able before to reach such intimacy and authenticity and therefore had never before noticed what kind of hearts beat inside certain "characters" and what minds can imagine other worlds.

This concerns all group members, obviously, the more so depending on how little they knew their original human nature, when they had a habit of considering themselves "a badly grown plant", "a freak", "a dumb brother", "an unwanted child", "an ugly duckling", "a black sheep", "a pervert", "a sleeping beauty", and many more sentences, prophecies, and Scripts that had come true and consolidated in the previous years of their life.

They are so surprised at finding so much beauty in themselves and in the others that they are moved by the "destiny" of all.

Slowly, under our joyful and surprised eyes it seems that something more is happening than just a new blooming of life; I think it is a reconciliation with the human species.

If this is not learning how to love, considering how imprecise this word is, it is certainly something very similar to it, maybe we can call it human sympathy, compassion, understanding, tolerance, and maybe we could even say "communion", all words that should be interpreted in their original meaning.

But maybe what happens could be more scientifically called a revitalization of the BELONGING drive typical of humankind that we always see in the affective attunement that we are able to build in many moments of our life.

And as we will see, even in painful situations.

## Bibliography

Allemandri D., Baldacci M., Ciurli M. P., Poidomani S., Procacci M. A., Salnitro P., (2012) *Bisogni spezzati, bisogni ritrovati. Nuovi orizzonti di analisi transazionale elaborati nella bottega di Carlo Moiso* (*Broken Needs. Rediscovered Needs. New Horizons of Transactional Analysis Developed in the Workshop of Carlo Moiso*). Roma, Alpes.

Berne E. (1961) *TA in Psychotherapy*. New York, Grove Press.

Berne E. (1966) *Principles of Group Treatment*. New York, Oxford University Press.

Cosso A. (2014) Copione, narrazione, destino, identità, storytelling (Script, narrative, destiny, identity, storytelling). In *RIC Rivista Italiana di Counseling*, 1(1).

Dehaene S. (2014) *Consciousness and the Brain: Deciphering How the Brain codes Our Thoughts*. New York, Viking Press.

English F. (1992) *Analyse Transactionnelle et Emotions*. (*Transactional analysis and emotions*). Paris, Desclée de Brouwer.

Goulding R., Goulding M. (1976) Injunctions, decisions, and redecisions. In *Transactional Analysis Journal*, 6: 41–48.

Goulding R., Goulding M. (1979) *Changing Lives Through Redecision Therapy*. New York, Brunner/Mazel.

Gregoire J. (2007) *Les orientations récentes de l'analyse transactionnelle* (*The new direction of transactional analysis*). Lyon, Les Editions d'Analys transactionelle.

Karpman S. (1968) Fairy tales and script drama analysis. In *Transactional Anayisis Bulletin*, 7(26).

Langer A. (1994) Quattro consigli per un futuro amico. (Four Tips for a Future Friend). In *Rocca*, 8-1995, Cittadella di Assisi.

Langer A. (2011) *Il viaggiatore leggero. Scritti 1961 – 1995* (*The Light Traveler*). Palermo, Sellerio.

Lowen A. (1975) *Bioenergetics*. New York, Coward, McCann & Geoghegan.

Magrograssi G. (2014) *I gioche che giochiamo* (*The Games We Play*). Milano, Baldini Castoldi.

Marchino L. (1995) *La bioenergetica* (*Bioenergetics*). Milano, Xenia.

Pagliarani L. (1985) *Il coraggio di Venere. Anti-manuale di psico-socio-analisi della vita presente.* (*The Courage of Venus. Anti-Manual of Psycho-Socio-Analysis of Present Life*). Milano, Raffaello Cortina.

Stewart I., Joines, V. (1996) *TA Today: A New Introduction to Transactional Analysis.* Melton Mombray, UK, Life Space.

Chapter 9

# The basic fault is the wound of non-loveRs

I. Yalom and M. Leszcz in *The Theory and Practice of Group Psychotherapy* wrote:

> In an outcome study, my colleagues and I demonstrated that group therapy patients, somewhere between the third and sixth month of therapy, often undergo a shift in their therapeutic goals. Their initial goal, relief of suffering, is modified and eventually replaced by new goals, usually interpersonal in nature. Thus goals changed from wanting relief from anxiety or depression to wanting to learn how to communicate with others, to be more trusting and honest with others, to learn to love.
>
> (1970, p. 19)

This is quite true; at the beginning we always agree with patients to a therapy contract that includes the first behavioral goals, modes, payments, rules, and so on, but in most cases the contract is only a way to clarify methods and limits of the intervention.

Then what usually happens is that the true problems tend to surface when a certain degree of intimacy is reached and the patient starts to see their problems with a little more psychological and reflective competence.

Clearly the therapist's interventions affect this course and I, in particular, have the ambition to be helpful from the very beginning, but I also want to leave to the patient the widest possibilities not only to move in the direction they choose but also to share the modes of therapeutic work.

At times we focus on a specific behavior, at others they prefer that we listen to them because they need to lay down the burden of their suffering, or they ask for specific advice on sudden dramatic events. In sum, at the beginning, also in order to build trust and openness, we need to avoid directing patients too much and we should respect the requests they are able to make with their current awareness.

But, after a while, if there is enough availability, the deeper and more real motives of suffering, failure, loss, anger, and inadequate behaviors emerge.

DOI: 10.4324/9781003303831-9

Right below the water line of the ship battered by the waves of life we are able to see the ancient motives that started and supported their voyage, those behaviors and beliefs that "inevitably" led to choose a limited, unhappy, and unhealthy course.

Down there, as Yalom writes – but along with him I like to mention Balint's primary love (1985, 1992) and Schellenbaum's wound of the unloved (1990), on which the title of this chapter is modelled, and Stern (1995), Bowlby (1979, 1988), Mitchell (1988, 2001) and naturally Eric Berne (1961, 1966) and many transactional analysts like Karpman (2010), Steiner (1971, 1974) and others – we see emerge the most relevant because of the primary difficulty: to love and build relations from which one can obtain love and consideration.

When the elements constituting identity remain without basic acceptance, without loving exchanges, without proper recognitions, without OKness, this identity ends up being distorted, indistinct, incomplete.

Without the ability to establish loving relations, life is compromised and the other drives are deeply affected.

The basic sorrow is the one suffered with the very first relational figures and the ways to overcome it, the techniques and methods to contact and "conquer" it still have to be built.

In the past few years, I focused on this issue not because I had a sudden idea but because I realized that almost all my interventions led me in one direction: *to reactivate love toward one's parents.*

The final goal of my research appeared clearly after years of work, and it was to discover that as adults we do not need to be loved, we do not need recognitions or acceptance, but rather we need to reactivate our original love drive in a healthy and efficient way.

Some way or other we have had to restrain or freeze or distort our original drives oriented to realize our attachments; some way or other we have built our personal way to love, that mode has become the usual scenario of our love movies, our hard-wired default setting, as Foster Wallace called it (2009), our restrained Script, or our character armor.

In those early relations we have literally learned how to love and be loved and, if things didn't go well, it will be very difficult to change since we have been trained in that mode for years and in the end we convinced ourselves that we are made in that specific way and that the men and women we met in our lives we could only love (or not love) in that specific way.

I dedicated a whole chapter to the fragility of mothers in order for us to see them as sons and daughters and as therapists, or better as adults, with the compassion that children cannot possess.

This chapter more or less rewrites some papers I presented at congresses and some articles I published in various journals (Piccinino, 2011a, 2011b, 2012) and, as I said, represents the outcome of over 15 years of practice. The case histories I include obviously disguise the patients as much as possible, changing names, professions, and locations so that not even the patients can recognize themselves.

As I said above, persons come to therapy with the life conditions they managed to realize and with a given awareness of themselves and given abilities: they are sad, angry, depressed, confused, frozen, agitated, scared, insecure, but inside their suffering they hide a strong wish to love. It seems incredible that however denied and distorted for years, this drive still tries to realize itself.

The love drive in fact is surprisingly strong, as much as the drive to survival so that they often coincide like in the first months of life.

We should be able to take our patient's hand with love and tenderness; we need to welcome them, listen to them and make them feel that they can still find love.

Under the ashes of one's failures, the primordial fire still glows and burns, and if it could not burn in childhood, with the due differences, it can be rekindled now.

I describe below the seven steps for a therapy to regenerate the loving drive as I applied them in these years, retracing them along a case history taken as an example.

It is a reinterpretation of the well-Known Parent Interview described by McNeel (1976).

In summary this journey aims to:

- Reconsider the primary scenes where the injunction to "not love" was internalized and the loving drive was reduced or deviated
- Re-live the seasons in childhood and adult age where patients applied their personal freezing of their hearts.
- Reactivate the love drive returning with the mind to the moments when it was mortified
- Reanimate trust in oneself and recover the capacity for love

From a methodological point of view, this intervention requires a deep knowledge of the patient, a strong alliance and a clear contract, and therefore the patient's well-grounded capacity to trust.

It cannot be done at the beginning of therapy or with persons unwilling to perform regressive or emotionally laden work.

We know that any aborted effort at applying a technique produces a certain amount of frustration and an unpleasant sense of failure; however, if we apply it, it is because we reasonably foresee to succeed.

Below I describe the seven steps we made in an intensive group made up of 15 persons to whom I suggested a guided fantasy that could evoke childhood scenes concerning their loving relationship with their mothers.

At the end of the fantasy with each of those who were willing, we tried to understand what had emerged and what we could do on their love modes.

This does not mean that this technique cannot be used also during normal group psychotherapy or individual psychotherapy – on the contrary – but in those cases it is better to start from the material brought to sessions by the patient and later suggest to recall some past situation related to events of the present.

So one can start in different ways, but the activity should always aim at letting re-emerge from implicit memory an important situation of the past that exemplifies a negative adaptive decision repeated and confirmed in time.

The experience evoked, in fact, rarely relates to a single instance, as in the case of a single trauma, but in most cases, it is one of the many situations that a child had to suffer repeatedly and for a long time.

The episode that is remembered at the start is a single scene but, in the same session or later in the course of therapy, the constants of the relation will emerge: the mother's usual attitudes and the child's defensive responses that have become scripts.

The next step consists in connecting the adaptations made as children with the current behaviors that are their outcome.

I present only a few sentences for each step, leaving aside some on my initial interventions that always aim at explaining the procedure, establishing a contract for the session, giving explanations and so on. A precise description of the method would take much more space.

---

### 1st step

| | |
|---|---|
| 1st step: | **guided reflection to recover the caring mode of the parental figure and defensive response of the child that become, or will become in time, a script** |
| 2nd step: | description of the old experiences |
| 3rd step: | link with present life |
| 4th step: | impersonate mother |
| 5th step: | explanation of current modes |
| 6th step: | revaluation of love for mother |
| 7th step: | concrete change goals |

---

The final goal is obviously different from one person to the other, but in this phase the goal is common: we need to be aware of our reaction faced with mother's specific loving mode, of how one behaved with that kind of care, what one defensively decided to do of one's original drive that, let me remind you, in a newborn is basically trusting and vital, welcoming and altruistic as much as self-centered.

Here we see the meeting of two persons driven by two very powerful loving propensities, but one of the two, that still has a pure and uncontaminated drive, must adapt to the mother's modes in order to secure care and survival.

I include below some excerpts of the guided reflection proposed to a group. Before starting, group members performed relaxation exercises, which can vary in duration and intensity, in order to focus on their internal world.

Imagine a situation where you are very young, you are alone, mother is not there, she left for a while, for one or two days you are without her and you remember her face, her normal way of being. What do you feel during her absence? Do you miss her? A lot? A little or not at all? What emotions or feelings do you have? What thoughts do you have? Time passes and she is not back; do you miss her? How do you miss her? Is it nostalgia? Are you with other family members in this period? If yes, how do you feel with them? Are you happy all the same or do you miss her so much that it hurts? Try to remember a similar situation if it happened to you or imagine how it would have been, had it happened. You are a child alone, how do you feel without mother? ... Then at last they tell you that mother is coming back soon, what is your first reaction? And when she comes to the door, what do you do? What happens? Imagine a scene that could have happened when you were a child, how do you see it? How would you have been and how would she have been? Describe mentally that meeting as you remember it, if you remember anything similar or imagine what could have happened. And now imagine, if you haven't already done it, that when she comes home you run to her with your arms open, full of enthusiasm and joy, and you want to give her all your love; imagine smiling, calling her and hugging her, you are four or five. Is it something you would do? Or is it something you never did? What would you feel like doing when she comes back from an absence? If you think you could go and hug her, how does she respond to your offer of love? How do you find her, how does she respond, how does she behave? Mentally describe her attitude. See how it feels, what emotions you feel at her response, what happens to your enthusiasm, how do you respond in turn?

At the end of this reflection all members are invited to open their eyes and to think of the scene.

I ask what images were evoked by the loving relation between a member and their mother.

What struck them most and what they relived.

Whoever wants is invited to come near the therapist and talk.

At times someone is already crying and I get near and stay near waiting for that person to talk.

---

**2nd step**

| | |
|---|---|
| 1st step: | guided reflection |
| **2nd step:** | **description of the experiences induced by the guided reflection and awareness of how the person reacted in the past also toward the parent** |
| 3rd step: | link with present life |
| 4th step: | impersonate mother |
| 5th step: | explanation of current modes |
| 6th step: | revaluation of love for mother |
| 7th step: | concrete change goals |

---

In this phase, with great caution and giving plenty of time, I help members verbalize what they remembered during the guided reflection. I have a precise goal: to highlight what happened, responses, decisions, interrupted gestures, Injunctions acquired and Drivers enacted in those situations.

From then on it will be possible to go back and face the current Script.

The first person coming near who wanted to face his relation to his mother I called Duilio, the name of an Italian boxer famous in the 1950s (Duilio Loi), a fighter with a strong defense and a good taker.

I will describe my 7 steps with him, describing also some of my interventions. Here some relevant initial exchanges.

Of the scene you describe I remember only that when my mum left I was happy. When we were together she always ended by hitting me. I don't remember anything else, she yelled at me, thrusted forward like a fury. I stayed there and took all in without running away or responding; I protected myself as I could but I never cried. When I was 12 I learned how to give her some drops, as the doctor had taught me, without her seeing, so she would fall asleep. When she wasn't there it was a relief.

I was always alone and I went to the boardwalk and looked at couples snogging. I was different from the other boys, I never felt like playing or laughing. I tried to stay away from her, I was afraid of her and somehow disgusted by her, she was so vulgar! When it was possible I went to a neighbor's house, it was quiet there. I never looked her in the eyes, if I did she got angry and yelled "What are you looking at? Stop it!" I tried to pretend that she wasn't my mother. I couldn't possibly have run to her and hugged her. I can't imagine what would have happened.

I never did. And now ... I am still like that, I am a bear, also with my own children ...

---

**3rd step**

1st step:      guided reflection
2nd step:      description of the old experiences
**3rd step:    link the experiences from the guided reflection with present life
               and how the person activated his love relations from then on**
4th step:      impersonate mother
5th step:      explanation of current modes
6th step:      revaluation of love for mother
7th step:      concrete change goals

---

In this phase, the intervention aims at seeing how the person learned to love, repeating the modes experienced with his mother. Modes are never the same, obviously, the Script changes when one grows up also due to the presence of other figures, but some features are set as they have been felt and memorized.

We therefore have to find out which ones are relevant.

It is also very important to make clear that from then on the person has loved (or not loved) first of all his mother, affecting in turn his relation to her: the disappointed becomes disappointing, the non-loved becomes non-loving.

This is a crucial passage to offer to patients because, when they have been abused as children, they tend to consider themselves as innocent victims when adults and find it hard to see how they have participated for a long time and unconsciously in crystallizing a certain kind of relation. The loving drive that originally is authentic and trusting is overturned and becomes structured as the person repeats those distorted gestures in all his later significant relationships.

The aim of this step is also to let the person see the difference between his original way of loving and his current one, how he became with the persons he is currently meeting and with his mother, denying, first of all to himself and then to her too, a filial love that is inescapable even if in quite different forms.

The person has to see that his mode has been insufficient or disappointing, violent or cruel or distancing.

Duilio is not the "non-loving that needs to heal"; he is the one who has to stop recriminating and asking others what he in the first place (or better in the second) has no longer been able to give.

Here are some of Duilio's reflections that I slowly help to emerge:

I even married one day and had two children but I have always been passive. I understood recently that I did nothing to build a decent relation, to get what I needed. But at the time I knew nothing of my needs. The relation to my wife wasn't so bad, but she started cheating on me and I pretended not to see, I just kept silent, she told me a lot of lies at the time. Now it seems impossible but I thought that a guy like me did not deserve anything better. I did all she told me to be a good husband and a good father: I worked, ran errands, drove her and the kids where they wanted to go. They had all the material things they needed and I never complained. I am good at being at the service of others. Then after cheating on me, she even left me and I left her everything, the flat and even the kids.

From then I only have lovers in other cities. But I keep them at a distance; I go and see them in the weekends. The last lover I had lived in France. I spent a lot of money on airfare and hotels but it was OK with me. I got some loving and sex but then at home I felt lonely. When I am alone at home I surf porn sites and masturbate until I am exhausted.

While Duilio talks I make some connections. For example, I make him notice that he already had said that as a boy he would go and look at couples snogging.

It's true! It's like you say and now I understand, I still look at others having sex as I did as boy when I went to look at those who parked on the board-walk, I masturbate, I comfort myself, I feel like shit. But why do I feel like shit?

This question deserves a clear and strong answer but offered with warmth and understanding because he needs to be brought back to his responsibilities in life, so I say something like:

You feel like shit because from then on you stopped loving, and one cannot live without love, sexual enjoyment without any form of affection is only temporary and worsens the situation because it just stresses what is lacking. So you repeat a behavior that does not meet your wish for love, even mastur-bation never leads to meeting your need for love. So distant lovers are just an effort at protecting yourself from the risks of intimacy and closeness that you have always been afraid to build. And so your life is made of peaks and troughs and how can you go on like this?

The answer is that to stop loving really hurts, dehumanizes and makes us feel empty and useless.

---

**4th step**

| | |
|---|---|
| 1st step: | guided reflection |
| 2nd step: | description of the old experiences |
| 3rd step: | link with present life |

| | |
|---|---|
| **4th step:** | **impersonate mother in relation with her child son and let emerge her impossibilities and limits and her underlying love. Highlight how the love drive has not been seen (or has been forgotten) by the son due to the overpowering and constant frustration received but also to his defensive responses** |
| 5th step: | explanation of current modes |
| 6th step: | revaluation of love for mother |
| 7th step: | concrete change goals |

This is a very delicate phase because it consists in letting emotions and behaviors registered by the scared child emerge as they were felt at the time.

Many "negative and defensive" decisions taken by the child were enacted in a state of fear and exhaustion.

At that age a child is defenseless and unable to make sense of what is taking place.

They always come to catastrophic and scary conclusions

To return to primary scenes of this type aims at analyzing them today in a novel way, more complete, more truthful, discovering their meaning, clarifying their historical motives, understanding better what was going on and in the end trying to reevaluate the mother's figure for what is possible because, as I tried to explain above, her destructive intentions were only involuntary.

I always salvage the underlying maternal or paternal love drive distinguishing it clearly from their crazy or manic behaviors.

To make the patient impersonate the mother and not consider enough their narrative or other techniques such as the "parent interview" (McNeel, 1976) has the clear advantage of making explicit the emotional content that inevitably carries along forgotten expressions and involuntary contents that at times turn out being extremely relevant.

The core experiences introjected as children and stored in implicit memory, once triggered into full expression, almost always unleash new and deeper emotions and memories that at the time had made such an "impression" that they had become some sort of script commands, although repressed, due to the huge emotion involved, in this case fear.

So I ask Duilio to impersonate his mother when she was screaming and hitting him.

He accepts, although with great suffering, and I tell him that those voices "must" come out if they are still inside him hurting him.

I build an adequate setting with him and I help him identify in his mother and I invite him to address his child self, as if he were standing there in front of him.

I am close to him and at times I put my hand on his back, in a way I am close to his mother and if it is true that I am inviting "her" to let out the worst in herself; it is also true that I am helping "her" to lay off the load of her actions, at last confessing her anxiety and tragic difficulty in being a mother.

I take for granted that it is awful for a mother too not to be able to love her child, not to take pleasure from this relation.

And now Duilio must know what actually happened to his mother to have treated him that way.

Now the patient will get in contact with the emotional and behavioral world of his mother (or father in other cases), will enter the enormity of her "tragedy" and instead of suffering as the victim, he will feel what happened inside her, what made her act like that.

Duilio-mother starts with slurs and swear words, there is more desperation than anger and I invite him to raise his voice and yell the slurs until I hear a deformed and terrifying voice that insults her son, tells him he is good for nothing and always stares at her with his imploring eyes. "What do you want from me? Piss off!" he screams and shakes while I invite him to say all that comes to his mind. Then, when I think enough anger has been vented, I ask her to explain herself to that child, to tell him what happened and why she is so upset and angry at him and what she wants from him. She cries that her life ended with the death of her mother who died when she had already left home to study and work as an apprentice in a shop in the nearest big city. She managed to leave home at age 15, running away from a large family, very poor and rough, farmers who treated her mostly with slurs and blows.

When she moved to the city she spent a wonderful year working as milliner for high society ladies right after World War II but when her mother suddenly died, she had to go back home to help her father raise her younger siblings.

And that was to go back to hell.

As soon as she could, she married the first guy she had met, but when Duilio was born she fell ill, of nerves, she says.

And she locked herself in due to a "mental breakdown".

They all want something from me, I can't do it anymore, you took my life, you too, you want me always with you and look at me as if I was crazy with eyes like a beaten puppy, what do you want from me!?

But after vomiting her desperation for her life she adds something unexpected:

But I wanted you to study, to be a good boy so that you could leave this shithole. And instead you are still here, wondering and doing nothing, good for nothing, like my father, like your father! And like my husband, you men are assholes! And I must serve you all, what men are you? What are you looking at? Why do you stare at me, you pig. I am not yet dead!

Unlike with other techniques, here the therapist does not ask for information but helps the patient "hear again" his mother's words, relive her emotions that here are anger and pain, that he heard as a child and stored, in part buried in his unconscious and implicit memory.

It is evident in these cases that our first experiences are stored in our memory in neuronal circuits that keep information important for our lives.

For young Duilio the fear of closeness is the strong and understandable permanent outcome of this relation, just like his adaptive response from Strong to Pleasing to Submitted.

The reemergence of the actual experience that created his script Is what will help him understand with an open heart the tragedy he happened to be born in, his loving responses, his passivity and his compensatory sexuality.

---

**5th step**

| 1st step: | guided reflection |
|---|---|
| 2nd step: | description of the old experiences |
| 3rd step: | link with present life |
| 4th step: | impersonate mother |
| **5th step:** | **explanation of current modes, collection of information emerged and explanation of the current way of loving. Analysis of the loving Script: Injunctions, Drivers, Opinions, Decisions, etc. Re-evaluation of mother's love and impossibility for both to be different at the time** |
| 6th step: | revaluation of love for mother |
| 7th step: | concrete change goals |

---

At the end Duilio, exhausted, collapsed but during the scene he had also remembered a detail that shook him deeply: his mother had always incited him to move, to study, to leave. And in fact he had moved to the city, the same city his mother had moved to, and he was the only one in the extended family who had graduated from university.

So I ask him to change place, to put himself in between mother and son. This is the moment of reflection for the Adult Ego State, for today's Duilio, no longer a scared child. I ask him what he thinks of this and this is his reply:

> But then she wanted me to be saved! And I followed her advice, I did what she had done!

He looks at me, stunned, and I tell him that he did even more: he completed his mother's journey to the city, he made his mother's dream come true.

> So, if I graduated and moved to the city I owe it to her too, gosh I never thought about it! And if she failed it wasn't her fault, she had to go back to

the village to raise her siblings. It must have been awful for her to come back. Poor mummy! That's why she then had a psychological breakdown. That's why she had such a fear of links and was unable to create different ones.

Even with her, I never learned to build a relationship, I didn't even know one could love actively. I kept going to see the others making love on the internet! Poor mummy, poor me! Even now that she needs me I flee her, I didn't even try to change our relation, maybe trying to find a different way of being together. I never felt compassion for her! But now I do pity her!

And here Duilio starts crying, big tears falling from his eyes, but he is crying because he feels compassion for his mother, for her madness, that had net even been treated properly by doctors at the time, for his absent father, always working and totally unable to manage that crazy, fat aggressive wife. Duilio cries for his life too.

Then he starts understanding that his way of loving his wife and children was a reaction to the way of loving of his mother, that it is her same way of loving, becoming the one who continues, until now totally unaware, his mother's and his family's script.

It should also be noted that his father too was a simple and rough person, the type that spends his whole time working, spending little time at home and unable to build warm relations with his children. And often he came home already drunk. Then he fell seriously ill and in the period Duilio relived he was constantly in bed, semiconscious, and cared for by his wife.

Duilio's belonging drive had been deeply compromised, as I said, even before this episode and we can well imagine it, because his mother had been under constant drug treatment.

The messages he had received from his mother were do not love, do not feel, do not be important, do not be intimate, with the ensuing drivers to be Strong, Please, and Try Hard in any way to obtain a minimum of acceptance.

It was unthinkable for him to imagine that he could be lovable and loving just how he was.

Everything needed to be earned.

At a more general level we should never forget that a detached child always sends signals of indifference to their parents and to others, thus feeding a climate of coldness which is the last thing they need.

So Duilio organized his loving relations; he had become aloof and made do with little solitary and temporary pleasure or sexual intercourse every two months.

Let me remind you, as I mentioned above, that many mothers realize that their children have disinvested them very early on and that basically they are physically and affectively detached.

Many of them say they felt rejected and powerless and therefore stopped trying to get in contact again.

This pains them but they are unable to explain it, if not with the fact that this is their child's "nature".

It is clearly difficult for them to assume the heavy responsibility of their children's lack of affection and to be able to ask themselves why their child does not look for them anymore.

Since they are not aware of their own lack of affection, they end up stopping to try to solve this and become even more passive, as per their Script.

The internalized detachment from one's mother becomes also an intrapsychic detachment from parts of oneself: those who did not internalize a good Parent lack an internal loving warm attitude toward themselves.

They cannot care for themselves, understand their needs, so in TA we talk of an excluded Affective Parent to indicate the structural absence of parts loving toward oneself, and in fact for Duilio it was especially hard to understand how much he needed a closeness that he had never had.

His loneliness, his endless working, his affective distance from his wife and his children, his merely operational presence, his divorce, his masturbation were inadequate responses to what he had always lacked.

When he felt lonely he masturbated to fill his affective void, just like a bulimic person introduces food to fill their affective void.

Had he remained how he was when he came to therapy, Duilio would have never been able to feel how huge his lack of love was as it was substituted by work and a deviated sexuality; his need for love was truly difficult to feel.

Beyond an occasional anxiety and an inexplicable constant distress, he felt that his suffering wasn't so bad and he managed almost "well.

With these premises it was impossible to look for what he needed.

The internalized overpowering wound of the "non-loving" made it very difficult to build new and healthy loving relations, it stabilized a Script of solitude and lack of love that obviously blocked him from trying to find in adult life what he had never "found" in childhood.

A last consideration to close this step concerns the limited perceptions of children in conditions like the ones we described here: once mother is perceived as an "enemy" or as dangerous, it will be difficult for the child to give value to the care he probably received, the sacrifices made, the nourishment and all the positive actions that must have been done if we have in front of us a lively and active person, despite his wounds and lack of love.

Duilio was however a clever and nice man, had a good sense of humor, he was aloof but was always available and soft.

And in fact it always happens that a patient after the kind of work I described, when they start seeing their mother with different eyes, suddenly remember the positive attitudes of their parents that they had totally forgotten.

I remember a young woman who during a seriously regressive exercise had suddenly remembered her mother giving her a bath when she was about two years old!

That image, although actually experienced, had been forgotten for over 30 years, suffocated as she was by her mother's other frequent inadequate attitudes.

Only in that moment, thanks to a certain reconciliation with the past, a situation and an emotion had resurfaced putting her mother, always considered in negative terms, in a new light.

That tenderness, care, physical intimacy had existed and, when it was remembered, had become a new emotional and behavioral internal resource for that woman.

From that moment on the patient's gaze was no longer satisfied with the good/bad mother or friend/foe dichotomy that had been useful to differentiate and defend herself, but recovered and felt again with great thankfulness the few moments of peace, care, intimacy or happiness.

To discover that one has had a mother that was also "good" emerging from a forgotten past (a mother that can be internalized and become a part of herself, loving and generous) is an indescribable relief, like being freed from a shameful original sin and to find herself innocent again and willing to love.

---

**6th step**

| | |
|---|---|
| 1st step: | guided reflection |
| 2nd step: | description of the old experiences |
| 3rd step: | link with present life |
| 4th step: | impersonate mother |
| 5th step: | explanation of current modes |
| **6th step:** | **revaluation of love for mother, transformation of the relation, return to living one's original love drive and change one's affective pattern of relating learned and suffered. "But today ... can you love a mother like yours?"** |
| 7th step: | concrete change goals |

---

As I was saying in the previous chapter, if the affective damage is deep and early, it certainly derives from the primary relation with the mother in the first years of life, and it is with her that one should recover it. It is also a problem that concerns the structure of personality: the Child part is depressed as a whole with deep damage to the capacity for feeling and the propensity to love.

But now Duilio is allowed to feel, love for his mother has been recovered, reconciliation is near thanks to the discovery of her "good" part and to a deeper knowledge of reality.

Mother is now quite different, more similar to the real one, more complete, she gave what she could and she is in this case heroic and tragic, at the same time victim and persecutor.

This new mother is a woman collapsed inside her Script that is also a social, family and gender Script that for a short time had seemed to allow her a way out by making her flee to the city. But she is also a mother that, despite her madness, indicated to her son a way to salvation, the same she had not been allowed to follow.

Duilio, thanks to his parents, had been able to study and move to the city, his mother had not been allowed to do it. In this phase I help Duilio redefine his way of loving first of all his mother and the question I ask while he is feeling a pure, intense and deep, ancestral, and "instinctive" emotion is pronounced in a solemn way,

"But today, can you love a mother like yours?"

In front of the whole group Duilio broke into tears "for" her and her fate, for what his mother suffered in a life much worse than his. He then recovered and said:

> I feel like one who has to learn to love from scratch; no that's not exactly true, my poor mother had lived her whole life on drugs but she cared for me, for what she could, now I feel that I too loved her for what I could. She gave me life and then pushed me more or less unawares to leave the place where I was born. Now I want to get also my children back, even if I feel that my attraction to them is still feeble. I understand that I must not leave them alone with their mother anymore, even if this is more sense of duty than love. And so I ended up doing like my father who was never there for me.
>
> Now that I met a woman here in this city, maybe I can start looking for her although she seems even more scared than I am. I am the one who wants to love her. I am a beginner, I know, I have to get out of the passivity that made me stay there and let myself be beaten without feeling anything. I have to learn not to be afraid of being close; I want to have a free heart and offer my love. No longer an onlooker.

The mother's love that had been forgotten needs to be revaluated, but also the son's love should be reaffirmed, so I made Duilio think of the great love act that he did when he remained and let himself be beaten without reacting.

He could have hit his mother when he was older but he never did; he could have given her more drops and killed her.

An act of love was also the care he provided her and that too he remembered with great intensity because from a very early age he had become her doctor. He was even able to give her a massage after the angry fits that left her exhausted so that numbed by her medicine she would doze off.

I want to add that this 6th phase is innovative and "demanding". In fact, often psychotherapists and patients consider an intrapsychic change sufficient or find it enough to apply the new decisions only to new or existing couple relations, leaving the relations with the actual parents untouched.

I can't say that it is possible to do this every time (I think of cases of rape, for example) but I think that changing how one concretely loves their parents is crucial for reaching a complete and deep pacification with the story of one's life.

In any case, in my experience if one rediscovers a good mother, the love drive toward her is immediately reactivated; to go and care and help materially one's parents is a finishing line for anyone's life course.

It is not so much the will to make peace or forgive but rather the rediscovery of the hidden part of our parents that we can at last love and of a part of ourselves that had not been able to offer them all our loving potential.

It is not a moral acquisition, it is a way of thanking them for the life we received, recognition and thanks for the hours of sleep lost, the time and effort they dedicated to their children. It is also a way to make amends for many years of distance and flight and the subsequent feelings of indifference, bad moods, disappointment, or hatred.

Even if they had told us, how often unfortunately happens, to unburden themselves of guilt, that they had wished to abort us or to abandon us, in the end they did not do it, love prevailed, they kept us and brought us to a sufficient degree of maturation so that we could live and wish to live happily.

We know quite well that even abandoned or adopted children always look for some form of rehabilitation of their parents.

How can we interpret this nostalgia, this wish to know, this effort at reconstructing an understandable and acceptable past, if not as the unquenchable need to find one's healthy and good roots, to tie again the thin but strong thread of a primordial love between children and parents?

That initial happiness, that pervasive and confused wellbeing, that totally trusting abandonment, those drives and those protected "landings" cannot be totally forgotten because we keep them in our hearts, bodies, skin, and this is how they can reemerge from implicit unconscious memory, those infinite joys can become the guiding stars that from now on can lighten our journey into love.

We often do not remember "cognitively" but we remember emotionally and bodily.

This is why the pursuit of happiness is inevitable also for those who seem cynical, pessimistic and defeatist.

If we want to help our patients to reconstruct self-esteem and serenity, if we want to help them be at peace with themselves and the world and, in the end, to love, we must always favor the elimination of any original sin that can trouble their heart and journey.

Our identity is made of the story we tell ourselves and our OKness will depend from it.

But it is also inevitable to become parents of our parents; it is one target in our life course: they age and we become adults, we will do what we can for as long as we manage, for what our life activities allow, but if we don't succeed not so much to forgive their errors but to love and accept them as they are, we will never learn compassion neither for them nor for our limits nor for those of others.

We are born Child, then we should become (also and mainly) Adults and in the end Parents. I find that it is against nature not to "honor" those who gave us life only because they also made us suffer, just like against nature is not to love our children only because they are not like us or because we don't like them that much.

---

### 7th step

| | |
|---|---|
| 1st step: | guided reflection |
| 2nd step: | description of the old experiences |
| 3rd step: | link with present life |
| 4th step: | impersonate mother |
| 5th step: | explanation of current modes |
| 6th step: | revaluation of love for mother |
| **7th step:** | **re-experience the reactivated drive with mother, other family members, partners, children, the therapy group, the therapist. Establish concrete supervised goals to learn again the capacity for love. Remember that the love drive is original and a condition for the survival of adults too** |

---

The last step completes the work and transfers it to everyday life starting from the relations with parents.

In an evolutionistic perspective we cannot forget that each one of us came to life "thanks" to parents that cannot but be themselves, the outcome of a specific humankind that is historically, psychologically and anthropologically typical of that section of evolutionary history where they happened to be born. In any case, they have decided to bring us to the world, take care of us and bring us exactly to that point of "maturation" where they were at the moment of our birth, with that culture, that phase of human evolution, those limits, that madness, that availability and that capacity for care.

Children when small see what they can of all this, in most cases they know nothing of their parents' problems and realize that something is not coming and feel distressed so then they recriminate or become angry or leave or become passive, so they structure their Script and formulate some ideas that are however always partial.

I think that a good definition of Script could be the following: a system of life assumed to avoid the risk of feeling again the fundamental pain felt when our vital drives have been rejected.

In the case of the propensity to belonging, "I might be cold, detached, abusive, distant, violent and so on, but I will not risk again to offer my love and create an attachment and be rejected".

The adult person needs now to reflect about what they had decided at the time and ask "Do I still want this? Will I remain at the level of evolution my father and my mother led me to? What is the developmental passage I should make now?"

Our parents take us there, then we should decide where to go; we cannot complain too much, it has been like this for everybody and it always will be, even though someone is born in a luckier crib.

And this will happen to our children too.

Each person (therapists too) has a task in life, those of us who are lacking in love (or some other natural propensity to knowledge, self-realization or survival) due to the lacks of our parents, those of us who have understood this thanks to analysis, from now on have a magnificent task: to make our species progress, go beyond that limit, open that Script that mortifies us in our human prerogatives and at the same time undermines our happiness and completeness as human beings.

This is the flag we should post in front of our door.

So now Duilio holds his flag and fights – can we say it? – for a better world, for the world he should have met in the first place. He is no longer a victim of this world but its builder and co-creator.

Here is the summary description of his new love life, these are his contracts for changing and learning, expressed in a later session to the whole moved and applauding group:

- To recover a lasting relation with my children and fight for them to be raised with my values and principles
- To negotiate assertively with my wife the time I spend with my children
- To write a letter to my children to explain why in the past years I have been a distant and cold father even if diligent. I must apologize and ask for understanding, I grew up in "hell", or maybe in "purgatory"
- Go and see other persons when I feel lonely and go out of the house instead of masturbating, not only to find company, but also to offer my renewed relational energy
- To visit my parents once a month and cuddle my mother, but also my father
- To be warm with my partner even if she sometimes wants to be on her own, I can always see friends
- Hug the other group members when I feel I should
- Stop thinking I am stalking my therapist when I call him at home

This fighter can no longer accept that his relation to those who generated him remains so thin and worn. He wants a different relation with his mother and father, he can no longer go and see them in their village only out of duty.

He can no longer wait for phone calls that blackmail him to go and celebrate a holiday, he can no longer forget that his father lives quietly but estranged from him nor that his mother has become an old fat resigned lady after so many years of medicines.

One day he felt the impulse to see them, he left early from work and drove to their place. When he arrived he hugged his mother in the kitchen then went to his father, who was dozing as usual while waiting for dinner.

Without a word he lay down near him, touched his forehead and without realizing it in a few moments was asleep. Tears were in his eyes when he woke up after an hour.

His father remained silent and still, maybe he did not understand what had happened but he certainly felt that new closeness, they smiled to each other and hugged, then all three sat to dinner with an odd good mood.

Then he returned home keeping his parents in his heart; he felt he loved them.

There must be no original sin inherited from one's family anymore, there's more than enough evil in the world, it is neither rare nor simple, it is casual and inevitable always present in our lives in all the corners of nature. That's the only evil that we must know how to accept and that will be discussed in the chapter entitled "Pain Feeds Joy".

In conclusion of this chapter, I want to recall that what we obtain with these techniques is mainly deep intrapsychic peace, possibly definitive: to find inside ourselves a "good origin", a good mother, a good father, to eliminates that sense of constant danger in our alarmed internal Child, detached always defensive, that for years has been suspicious of a world until then petrified in a dark, scary, and always impending gloom.

Something like a Saturn devouring his children at every turn, an Ogre or Witch Parent kept alive inside oneself.

This is the resurrection that restarts the lost love drive, the "dormant opportunity" described by Stanislas Dehaene (2014).

There has never been an original sin nor guilt for anyone, neither for the children nor for the parents.

The world is not as scary as the one the child Duilio had stored in his heart; not only it is not so scary, it cannot be so scary. Anyhow it is certain that for Duilio it will never be so scary again.

For many other persons with whom I worked in this way the outcome has been similar: each of them found a new love world to "co-create".

By loving their mothers and fathers again, they all were able to start again, like a true prince or princess, children of kings and queens, wretched and tragic at times, but they too with a life of sorrow and frustrations that can be understood and treated with compassion.

If for a child some experiences of their parents' life are totally unexpected and incomprehensible, for an adult they can only be seen as a painful stretch of the long journey of humankind. And they need to observe it with the certainty that if those same parents had been able to do it, they would have certainly changed it.

In any case, an adult can always be helped to welcome and accept what happened, even in a hard, hellish, dramatic scene they can discover how their resilience allowed them to grow and develop abilities that it would have been difficult to let out, qualities that today they can at last put at the service of their happiness.

Some wounds will always stay within us, but once we know their dramatic relevance and the specific reasons why they happened, we will be able to stop considering the whole world like we had perceived it at the time.

At times it will not be possible to love the hand that held the stick but at least we have objectivized, understood, and expelled it from ourselves, because we do not want to have anything to do with that past and we do not want to re-create it.

If one cannot love that hand, one can at least pity it and leave it alone.

I think this is the only way to learn how to feel compassion, in addition to indignation for certain human "follies".

To be in analysis, having been able to start and complete it, makes patients (and us therapists) in a way privileged persons: a totally different culture, at times thanks to those very parents, made possible the move that led us to understand and want to change.

At times they feel like miracles, at times it feels like the inescapable evolutionary course of Nature that in time protects, grows, improves our species and makes it strong, blooming and civil.

In any case, we are here to try at least to facilitate that course.

The recovery of the original love drive is contagious; when eyes are again brilliant, when smiles are more frequent, when kindness, affection, acceptance, OKness, and trust radiate "naturally", the world itself changes and clears up.

Each person becomes a gift, an offering of oneself for what one is.

Backs straighten up because dignity lifts them, looks become kinder, the wish to live runs free and the original offer of love crops up again.

We can go back to being "lovers".

So when this happens, something more than the recovery of love toward one's parents also happens, and the consequences are different: new couples form, children are born, couples resume lovemaking, unexpected admirers crop up, new homes are bought, some persons leave, others return, princes and princesses know very well what to do with that offer of love that is blooming inside them.

Life resumes.

But we must remember that all around this idyllic picture there are also difficulties: these therapies shake and revive the belonging drive but in our busy and materialistic, consumerist and non-loving society, that is more and more replete with single persons and single mothers, absentminded husbands, greedy and insatiable persons, we risk with our work to leave our former patients in greater difficulty and contradiction with their reference environment.

The primacy of love life for mental health and for the happiness of human beings is not part of our practical life habits but is a war that these persons want to fight.

The original love drive is not undifferentiated in humans; just like our hominid ancestors we know today that a human being can be our enemy; madness, greed, bullying, unwarranted aggression, exploitation of men by men are around and inside us.

But if we know how to love and live in harmony with ourselves, we are able to live with some enemy, provided we don't get caught in useless skirmishes and battles.

## Bibliography

Balint M. (1985) *Primary Love and Psychoanalytic Technique*. New York, Routledge.

Balint M. (1992) *The Basic Fault: Therapeutic Aspects of Regression*. Evanston, Illinois U.S. Northwestern University Press.

Berne E. (1961) *TA in Psychotherapy*. New York, Grove Press.

Berne E. (1966) *Principles of Group Treatment*. New York, Oxford University Press.

Bowlby J. (1979) *The Making and Breaking of Affectional Bonds*. London, Routledge.

Bowlby J. (1988) *A Secure Base: Parent-Child Attachment and Healthy Human Development*. New York, Basic Books.

Dehaene S. (2014) *Consciousness and the Brain: Deciphering How the Brain codes Our Thoughts*. New York, Viking Press.

Foster Wallace D. (2009) *This Is Water*. New York, Little, Brown and Company.

Karpman S (2010) Intimacy analysis today. The intimacy scale and the personality pinwheel. In *Transactional Analysis Journal*, 40(3–4: 224–242.

McNeel J. (1976) The Parent interview. *Transactional Analysis Journal*, 6, (1): 61–68.

Mitchell S. A. (1988) *Relational Concepts in Psychoanalysis: An Integration*. Cambridge, MA, Harvard University Press.

Mitchell S. A. (2001) *Can Love Last? The Fate of Romance Over Time*. New York, Norton.

Piccinino G. (2011a) Pulsioni innate e riconoscimenti, un contributo alla teoria del Copione. (Innate drives and recognition, a contribution to script theory). In *AT Rivista Italiana di Analisi Transazionale e metodologie terapeutiche*. xxx, n° 22/2010, Roma, Simpat.

Piccinino G. (2011b) We empowerment. In *Pagine Mida*. Milano, Fondazione Mida.

Piccinino G. (2012) La ferita dei non amaNti. (The wound of non-lovers). In *Neopsiche* N°12, Torino, Ananke.

Schellenbaum P. (1990) *The Wound of the Unloved: Releasing the Life Energy*. Dorset, UK, Element Books.

Steiner C. (1971) The stroke economy. In *Transactional Analysis Journal*, 1, 3.

Steiner C. (1974) *Scripts People Live: Transactional Analysis of Life Scripts*. New York, Grove Press.

Stern D. (1995) *Motherhood Constellation: A Unified View of Parent-Infant Psychotherapy*. New York. Routledge.

Yalom I., Leszcz M. (1970) *The Theory and Practice of Group Psychotherapy*. New York, Basic Books.

# Chapter 10

# Giving "weight" to father and mother

I think it is evident how these techniques can impact also the other members of a group and, maybe at this point, one can better understand that it is useful to go beyond individual therapy. But I want to stress that in all cases therapy should start with individual sessions that are indispensable for a good start and the creation of a relation of openness and trust. The following steps are obvious but I think worth remembering:

- A precise and detailed diagnosis
- An introduction to "emotional literacy" to help the person be aware of their situation
- A first agreement on "what needs to be done". The goals to be reached in the initial phase represent the psychological contract, the alliance aimed at a concrete and observable goal
- A clarification of working modes, how therapy takes place. We are talking of times, frequency, rules, payments, and so forth, that represent the framework of administrative rules for our relation
- First interventions aimed at clarifying the origin of symptoms locating them in a wider understanding of personality that explains their appearance and their negative effect on everyday life
- First interventions to alleviate pain, support motivation for therapy and stimulate trust in the developmental opportunities of each person

Usually, it takes months of individual therapy before we can agree on joining a group. There patients will be able to talk about themselves with a quantum of psychological knowledge and receive all the advantages of acceptance and support, they will practice, meet the great sorrows of their past, start to see and trigger new deep changes, and they will celebrate.

In-depth work typical of the most advanced phases of therapy (what we call "re-decision" and "de-confusion" in the following scheme and that are aimed to restructuring personality) concerns the unveiling of oneself and one's story within a new and different relation where at last the undone, unsaid, unfelt can be expressed, understood and accepted.

DOI: 10.4324/9781003303831-10

Through the knowledge of one's unacted drives (just like through the analysis of dreams, the understanding of unaware repetitions of current attitudes, the reading of the various transferences, etc.) we can let resurface the more or less willfully internalized limitations that we call negative Script.

I add that when we make this exciting work in a group, thanks to the various confrontations and the knowledge of the stories of others, all members start to understand the relevance of infantile functioning and how many beliefs on one's childhood were limited and partial.

They start to understand that human nature (and therefore theirs too) is quite different from what they had imagined within the limited possibilities they had imagined as children.

They start to understand that they had good reasons to become what they are as adults. Their being "strong", "pleasing", "hurried", "perfect", "always trying hard", their choice not to be themselves, does not depend on chance or even less nature, and even less it is their fault and unchangeable.

They certainly had good reasons to give up realizing their drives and now they can see those reasons, which were the most obvious response to the limitations and lacks of the environment in which they grew.

These are the realizations that, if not already "healing", certainly are already opening a new road to change:

- It is not by chance that I lived like this for such a long time
- My automatic negative behaviors are not natural
- It's not my fault if I turned out this way
- What has been altered or hampered in my nature can now be changed; now I can change

While we expose the family *culture* where they grew, we give value to the deepest *nature* of persons and elevate to sacred the essence of their being human.

No one forgoes feeling love and affection, sentencing oneslf to narcissistic isolation or paranoid aggression and to always unsatisfying elations, unless one felt the awful pain of not being returned one's love at the beginning of life.

If all surges are quenched or disappointed, how can one survive but by stopping all motions?

No one gives up self-esteem if not to defend oneself from a constant confrontation with a "dominant other" that makes one feel inferior in all contacts.

No one becomes evil and feels all other persons are potential enemies if not to defend oneself from a world that has been *truly* aggressive and violent.

If it is true that adaptive responses always derive from the child's subjective perceptions, although at times they are dramatized and experienced worse than they actually were; it is also true that those messages were sent and should not have been sent to have a healthy and happy growth.

All defenses become pathological when in their primary relations children are forced to give up important parts of themselves, like propensities, relative capacities and basic functions, although the ways in which this happens are as numberless as the relational situations any child is involved in.

It is not always a question of forgoing; there can be confusion, muddles, ambivalence, contradictory wishes and fears, exaggerations, violence, "psychological tricks", and therefore also constant clumsy and awkward efforts at being close that in the end prove unsatisfying.

Repeated failures in trying to be loving or loved, like "I wish I could but I can't" all the time.

In TA we call psychological games (Berne, 1964, Magrograssi, 2014) the traps that poison the life of persons who did not receive permission to offer and ask for love, all those more or less unconscious and implicit, sometimes funny at others dramatic efforts at getting closer in the hope of being considered.

But since these behaviors are hampered by a prohibition or by low self-esteem, they end up being clumsy, manipulating, aggressive. One plays the Persecutor in order be feared, another plays Rescuer in order to receive thanks, and another plays Victim in order to be pitied.

As all the other drivers (Please, Try Hard, Be Strong, Hurry, Be Perfect) also Psychological Tricks end up looking for love and consideration with specific behaviors that do not have much in common, even when they don't end badly, with a global acceptance of the person, with the recognition of their value as human beings.

They look for OKness and acceptance donning a suit they think is festive while it is the only one they have found in the family closet, they think it will help them find love and instead it only reinforces socially and superficially that type of behavior.

A sentence, and in the end a Script, to a life fossilized in a character that is always searching for something that with that behavior they will never find.

The many persons I worked with are a rather evident sample collection of failures that certain behaviors lead to; love cannot be obtained with a compulsive repetition of one's specialties, even when they seem like a good substitute for natural and healthy behaviors, but it can be obtained with an authentic and trusting offering of oneself and with one's industry given freely to the world while realizing one's talents.

I want to repeat, however, that all these descriptions of types and the efforts at describing human suffering according to categories and schemes (including mine) should always be considered as rough general indications, like a map seen from a faraway satellite.

We therapists need to come down to earth, walk along with our patients and get to know their words and their answers that were built during many years. Only in this way, with shared language, values and goals, we will be able to walk along with them and understand through what winding roads they came to their specific suffering and in the end identify possible alternatives for their lives.

Many have tried to do without maps but they are indispensable; the important thing is that they are used as examples of *one* possible description of life to suggest to them so that they can tell it in their own words.

Neurophysiologists explain that our mind is made up of millions of synaptic roundabauts that open to different exits, but we select a few, the most impressive ones, and neglect the others until they become useless.

Millions of pieces of ancient information affect what we feel because, for example, since we have always perceived an extrovert woman as invasive and dangerous, we relate her immediately, like in the past, to a feeling of fear and to thoughts of avoidance and flight behaviors.

Millions of privileged neuronal connections respond to our current experiences basically with those ancient childhood reactions that we have repeated for years.

To stop to be afraid of a relation with a woman only because she is felt as invading requires the acquisition of new information, requires that in that very moment a synapsis transfers the initial information toward an even older way, almost totally forgotten at the bottom of implicit memory, the way of curiosity for example.

That archaic memory is the True Self and is the original natural drive that said "you can get to know her" or better even told me I could love that type of woman.

The new route of the original love drive can be traveled only if we change the information that once settled in our mind, new explanations, new thoughts, new emotions are needed, like these, for example:

> she did not invade you because she thought you were powerless, she was close to you because she was afraid to lose you or that you could hurt yourself, like it had happened to her mother – for example – and you gave up not because you were powerless but you couldn't do otherwise, you were a child and thought this was the right way to do.

Now we can love because we have learned that we can decide the distance, we have understood that we have our own personality that should be asserted and completed, for example.

When we become adults, we can give ourselves permission to be ourselves, to put limits to the wishes of others, we can lead the game of closeness and distance according to our times and modes and at the same time find someone we can play it with without submitting to their will as we did in the past.

This work decontaminates the behavioral possibilities of the present from the invasion of automatic responses established in the past; it explains what present fear is justified only by the old experiences that enslaved us.

If he learns how to lead the game with his mother, his love drive will be reactivated forever by learning the power that could not have been exerted at the time, learning a new adult way of loving where autonomy is always indispensable along with belonging, that power that makes us say "We can be together also at my conditions, in a way that is fine with me too".

An invaded child that doesn't know how to love will not be able to reactivate their love drive fully if they haven't first cleared the scared resentment that is similar to a constantly blaring alarm, stuck deep in their emotional world and often forgotten.

Can I love a mother like her?

How can they meet a partner and get close and make love and let themselves go in their arms offering their life with that horror movie constantly running in their mind?

In that movie they did not exist as persons, they could not say "Now yes" or "Now no", they could only sneak away, stay as little as possible, feeling small, needy, and helpless.

Is it clear that in my example I am referring to a person suffering from an anxiety syndrome that will probably induce premature ejaculation or psychosomatic vaginismus?

How many persons have I met that were unable to build mature love relations because they had not completed the natural course of that primary love with their mother that had remained interrupted! That incomplete love holds a drawstring with the past; one does not truly become adult if that thread is still tangled around one's heart.

Where can we go if we are still fighting to be loved and recognized as we wanted or how we should have been loved by our parents or those we consider like them, just to repeat that tragedy?

We are still children who face life with an angry face and our head turned back, our heart hardened by the lost love.

A few days ago a friend sent me a note answering my condolence message for the death of his mother, a woman with whom he had always had distressed and stormy relations:

> I thank you for your closeness and the love I felt that nourished me in these monuments of intense feelings for the loss of a mother that in the past few months had been weak, fragile, totally dependent and defenseless and was the person and the mother she could have been. And she would look at me with the wide-open shiny eyes of a lost child I had never been able to see in her. I could reconcile with her.

I had in therapy quite a few women who were unable to get pregnant because their love relations with their own mother or with both parents was incomplete and once they felt pacified they could at last have children.

Just like I met quite a few men who did not want any children until they reconciled with their fathers and they too had been able to become parents.

In humans filial love is an "instinct" so strong and pervasive that it cannot be easily suffocated. One needs a pacification that frees from dependence or, if this is not possible, gives up forever to any hope if this is "truly" non-realizable.

But if this is the case, we should first analyze carefully also the son's responsibilities.

These are loves that cannot be cancelled, they can evolve and become complete thanking for the good one has received and changing the still lingering bad.

This is the only way to leave in peace, also well prepared for new loves because we can give to our parents what we now own.

But should we not do this also with adult loves?

As I already mentioned, however, in the cases described in this book this is the procedure to give at last the permission to love, but I don't want readers to believe that this is always possible.

At times to set a distance and get free from evil and noxious family relations is already a victory and it would be difficult to ask for more.

I think of persons abused in various ways, abandoned children, exploited children and I think in particular of those persons that despite their good intentions as adults are still treated by their parents as step-children or obstacles to their lives

In these cases, too, it's up to the patients to indicate to us the level of change they wish for and are able to reach, and we need to respect it.

I was truly surprised when I discovered that the fourth commandment of Christianity "Honor your father and mother" should have been translated differently: the Hebrew verb *Kappod* can also be intended as "give weight", "give importance" with an evident semantic shift (http://www.iperbole.bologna.it/iperbole/llgalv/iperte/comandamenti/comandamenti/quarto_comandamento.htm).

This is exactly what I aim to do with therapy: discover the role parents have had in giving life to a new creature, for evil but especially for good.

Just like maternal and paternal love is a physiological and natural psychic event, so is filial love.

They are both necessary attachments for human nature to survive; forgive my insistence.

For millions of years children have been born loving their mother and father, for millions of years (sane) fathers and mothers have loved their children, these loves must change but I feel that forgoing them is an act "against nature".

The mind needs really to be turned upside down to be able to give them up and, when it does, the "wound of the non-loveRs" remains there, deep in our heart to alarm us at any meeting, both if we succeeded in being cynical and disillusioned and if we maintained a quantum of humanity.

This is truly an original sin: not to love one's father and mother and not to love one's children for me are on the same level and are both against nature.

And if we cannot love our parents who had the merit of bringing us to life and we can't love them with all their faults and limitations, how can we truly love the Other from ourselves that will have faults and limitations too?

Do we think the husband or wife we marry has fewer faults?

And all the other persons we will meet? By loving our parents as adult children we complete the course for learning how to love that humans must follow starting from the undifferentiated symbiosis of fetuses: from undifferentiated and con-fused love, when we are not yet individuals, as soon as we are born we grow toward an exchange of unconditional love and then slowly we discover the Other, we evolve toward the plurality of love investments, toward the full responsibility for our emotions, thoughts and attachments.

As adults we discover conditional loves and how easy it is to lose them if we don't know how to love; later we will be able to unconditionally love our children, maybe even our life partners for all our lives.

All along this route love for our parents is often behind us, we know it's there even if we think we don't need it anymore, even if we are busy with other persons, that knotted thorny memory still affects our modes and intensity, our trust in fellow humans.

But our course in learning how to love does not stop, not even after we have children; it cannot end there because the love drive, like the propensity for survival, evolution and self-realization, does not stop at a given age, is not satisfied only with romantic love, a spouse, a family, for its own nature it is not limited to these kinds of love; our community also requests our love and we need it in turn.

So we have a propensity to love, in addition to our children, our grandchildren and the children of our friends, our community, the persons around us, the earth maybe, where we have lived and also the persons that brought us into the world, our ancestors.

We realize it may be a little late, unfortunately, when we are old.

I think that our course in learning how to love can reach even higher.

We will be complete when at last we love life, with its ups and downs, with its miseries, injustice, uncompletedness, when we reach the joy of living and being in the world as it is, with our own mistakes and those of our parents.

Do we think we are better than them?

We only try to make fewer mistakes and this is evolution.

Of this we are responsible, knowing them and the damage they did to us, knowing the mistakes their parents made and the damage they did to them, knowing our own and their qualities, ancient and more recent, we can progress some more, maybe it won't be much for us but we will leave a better world than the one we found.

It is very difficult to love life for what it is without loving our parents and what they are and have been, and vice versa.

Bert Hellinger (1998), a much discussed psychotherapist, inventor of family constellations, wrote:

> To honor one's parents is to love and accept them as they are, and to honor the earth is to love and accept the earth as it is, with life and death, health and illness, with a beginning and an end. This is a deeply religious act. In former times, we called this worship. It is the ultimate religious act, and we experience it as complete surrender, costing nothing less than everything. It is the surrender that gives all and takes all and takes all and gives all — with love.
>
> (p. 324)

Now I can confess it more openly, I had said at the beginning that these therapeutic passages are quite ambitious, they intend to stimulate when possible to go beyond forgiveness and the pacification with one's family, they intend to reach internal peace, acceptance of the world as it is, loving not only the others but life itself with its difficulties and pain.

They want to stimulate for what is possible a contemplative attitude where the only judgment can be "so is the world", "we are human beings".

The possible, and as I said rather ambitious, goal for good psychotherapy may be this making peace can be this making peace with the past and with ourselves, not only forgive from the vantage point of our knowledge and reconciliate. It is a lot more; it is loving life in its entirety.

For this reason the therapy group must become also the place of joyful creations, not only because we laugh and are merry but because it becomes the "here and now" where one can get to know the others, mutually fertilizing, where one can love the Other and realize one's personality also through suffering when necessary and through the recognition and acceptance of diversity.

Our journey, even if we don't always know where we are going, must be happy not for the future but for a now that must arrive as soon as possible:

> like a healthy child playing enthusiastically with a toy: seeing their joy someone could try to take the toy from them, but the child will start playing with another toy and so on until someone continues thinking, wrongly, that the child's happiness depends on the toy.

Once again virtue rewards itself because virtue is the realization of our drive nature.

A man "can and must" be happy only because he exists, to remain alive is a privilege and life is too short for us to be wasting time.

Without birth no one would have had this opportunity and our birth has three protagonists: ourselves, two parents and the species that evolves through them.

The happiness of being in the world cannot but include also "thankfulness" and – between us and Nature – there are always two parents.

And the certainty that we don't ever have to be alone.

The one that follows is a broad description of the course of a therapy and of the possible interventions. It is my elaboration of the scheme brought forward in the work of Carlo Moiso (Allemandri et al., 2012) and Michele Novellino (2014, 2016).

This too is obviously only a roadmap, then each person has their own route and anything can happen: steps intertwine, often we move forwards and then have to move back to return to issues that had already found a solution.

The substitution of old neuronal circuits with new ones requires that we go back and reconsider the ancient automatic responses that are still active.

Patients don't really like this because they feel they are receding or are stuck at one point, but it is useful to realize that the new behavioral patterns are never definitive and that the earlier ones, although we tend to use them less and less, will not disappear completely. They will linger there, at the bottom of our archaic past, to remind us we need to be alert and careful in our new way of living.

The scheme is often overturned by the fact that in groups all members see the work of others and at times they change even only by participating emotionally and cognitively to the therapeutic experiences of others, at times they have surprising insights and deductions that we don't even expect.

So all our schemes and our progressive strategies collapse under our eyes. Luckily.

## Summary Scheme of the Phases of Therapy

### 1st: Alliance

To build a relation of openness and trust, favor authenticity and motivation, identify a proper intersubjective distance for this initial phase. Unconditional acceptance. Clarifying operations by means of questions, confrontations, explanations, interpretations, and the like. Support interventions for reassurance and encouragement.

### 2nd: Contract

Activities aimed at realizing a first approach to the goals to be reached. Analysis of priorities and clarification of the relevance of problems and of the course of therapy. Explanation of the psychological concepts necessary for a good awareness of what we are working on. Give value to the person's capacities supporting a positive and accepting view of themselves. In general at this point a person can join a group.

### 3rd: Focused interventions for clarifying and developing the main functions

Increase awareness of oneself and of one's relations. Analysis of the relation between drives and present happiness, needs and obstacles, rules of life and possibility to meet needs, check abilities. Take responsibility for one's actions. Learn the language of emotions: clarifications and explanation of language as a realistic expression of oneself, proprioceptive and exteroceptive competence. Awareness of the parts of oneself and their possible integration. Activities aimed at developing expressivity, integration and consistency of the various functions of personality (Parent, Adult, Child). Develop weak functions and unexpressed resources. New decisions to overcome the impasse between the conflicting parts of oneself and new Permissions. Integration of the different parts of oneself and check the achievement of therapeutic goals.

### 4th: Structural interventions

Activities aimed at the reemergence of ancient messages excluded from initial awareness: regressions, guided fantasies, work on the body, psychodramatic techniques, and the like, to recover past experiences that favored negative adaptations and Script decisions and find new substitute solutions for the here and now. Expression of repressed and suppressed emotions. Discovery of new more realistic narratives of the past and corrective experiences related to the expected changes. Understanding of projections and transference identifications toward the therapist and other group members. Relive parental tragedies to understand them emotionally and turn them into history (the wound of the non-loveRs). Make peace with the figures of the past and recovery of all drives. Development of new capacities required for the realization of drives. Acceptance of oneself and consolidation of OKness.

### 5th: Training

Crystallization of considerations concerning the past and new behaviors to be strengthened. Application in the here and now, in the group and in public life, of new capacities. Periodic check of positive results, celebrations, positive recognitions. Enhancement of acquired abilities and check of the possibility that the persons can continue their journey on their own. Progressive separation based on the person's requirements and the actual stabilization of change, also in the light of events that could boycott change later on.

## Bibliography

Allemandri D., Baldacci M., Ciurli M. P., Poidomani S., Procacci M. A., Salnitro P., (2012) *Bisogni spezzati, bisogni ritrovati. Nuovi orizzonti di analisi transazionale elaborati nella bottega di Carlo Moiso* (*Broken Needs. Rediscovered Needs. New Horizons of Transactional Analysis Developed in the Workshop of Carlo Moiso*). Roma, Alpes Italia ED.

Berne E. (1964) *Games People Play*. New York, Grove Press.

Hellinger B. (1998) *Ordungen der Liebe* (*Orders of Love*). Heidelberg, Carl-Auer.

Magrograssi G. (2014) *I gioche che giochiamo* (*The Games We Play*). Milano, Baldini Castoldi.

Novellino M. (2014) *Seminari berniani. La prassi dell'analisi transazionale.* (*Bernian Seminars. The Praxis of Transactional Analysis*). Milano, F. Angeli.

Novellino M. (2016) *Psicoanalisi transazionale. Manuale di psicodinamica relazionale per psicoterapeuti e counselor.* (*Transactional Psychoanalysis. Handbook of Relational Psychodynamics for Psychotherapists and Counselors*). Milano, F. Angeli.

# Chapter 11

# Changing the past?
# Two examples

Although I have included a reconstruction of a phase of Duilio's therapy, I am not sure that this kind of therapeutic work is clear also to those outside the field. Luckily a few years ago a young therapist who had completed her personal group analysis with me asked me to continue for a few months as a silent audience in order to see how I worked "from the outside". In exchange for this, she recorded the sessions. So, after receiving the consent of all the patients in the group, we located her in a corner of the room where she could listen without participating and interfering with our work.

After a few weeks her presence was totally forgotten and I can say we worked as if she was not there. We had agreed that at the end of that period she would transcribe some sessions and include her comments.

Below I am including two examples of treatment. In italics are the words of the patients interspersed with my interventions and my reflections that explain their rationale.

The transcription is basically verbatim, except for a few changes introduced to make the different persons recognizable. I also made a few syntactic corrections to make the conversations fully understandable.

## First example: Giulia

This first fragment concerns a woman in her early thirties who is reaching the end of her therapy. So far she has overcome some relevant problems of identity and acceptance of herself. When she started treatment she also had rather heavy psychosomatic problems and lacked the ability to feel important and worthy of equal love relations.

Usually her love relations concerned persons that were more needy and distressed than her. At this point of her treatment she had stopped being the Rescuer (Karpman, 1968) and had established an important relation with a man, very warm and older than her.

She knows well her needs and limitations but is still affected by persisting insomnia.

DOI: 10.4324/9781003303831-11

The problem concerns her survival drive but also the belonging drive; since she still doesn't feel important enough, she finds it very hard to protect herself, she knows that some parts of her are still fragile, her body for example had become very rigid, especially her knees and back when she felt "great fears" and today she still cannot relax fully when sleeping and making love.

These moments require complex and heavy strategies that do not always work also because she cannot say explicitly what she needs.

In her story there is also a rather absent father, much devalued by her mother and always blamed for his and his family's problem, but most of all there is a mother who has always been very unhappy, anxious, and, as we will see, a cause of anxiety for her daughter.

Giulia is a beautiful young woman, clever, tall with beautiful blond hair and bright eyes full of life and at times of anxiety.

She dresses well although she is not rich but has a very feminine taste and often the other group members congratulate her for her looks.

At the beginning her image of herself did not correspond at all to her beauty and femininity.

Until the session we are going to describe group therapy had been quite satisfying also in concrete terms. In fact she managed to move out of her parents' home, find a job that supports her independent life and recognizes her professional talent and her beauty.

Her newly established romantic relation seems to crown the journey she made so far.

*GIULIA:*　　　*Last night I did not sleep again, I want to solve this problem; we have to return to my sleep. if I want to end psychotherapy I need to sleep well, I must.*

*TERAPEUTA:*　Yes, of course, what do you want to start with?

*GIULIA:*　　　*Here's what happened last night. At 10.30 Tobia and I go to bed to chat and cuddle but when I start sleeping, in the sense that I feel I am falling asleep, I put earplugs on and turn the light off I start feeling restless, my heart beats faster and sleep leaves me. From then on anything Tobia does bothers me, even his cuddles bother me, he says OK, let's not sleep, so I get closer to him, he cuddles me and I fall asleep but lightly. I woke at 4.30 for a bad dream. I remember that in the dream my mother kept berating me for how I organized my work life for the future and said: "But you haven't dome anything yet" and I didn't like this pressure, it was like saying that at my age other persons already have their life job while I don't.*

*TERAPEUTA:*　We could talk of the dream, but let's do this today (he takes a mattress and puts it in front of Giulia) come, lie down here, make yourself comfortable and take three deep breaths; when you inhale let the air go down deep in your belly, when you exhale let all the air out and relax. OK, that's good, now keep breathing regularly and do what I ask very slowly. To lie down helps you get in touch with yourself, with the feelings and emotions of yesterday, let your thoughts flow freely and then return to last night's situation when you let yourself be cuddled before sleeping. You are relaxed and ready to fall asleep.

> I know where I want to go with her, she is still very entangled in her relations, she still cannot choose to do what she wants; she often oscillates between what she wants to do and the fear of being a burden. I know her mother is anxious and Giulia has always found it hard to let go and until now even sexually this is not easy for her. What I want to do should help her relive last night's emotions. I use this technique often with this group and for Giulia it is nothing new. This is why I move so easily and without preparation.

*TERAPEUTA*: Are you ready? (She nods) OK, now you were thinking you were ready to fall asleep and unrest set in, go back to that moment ... when you have recovered the feeling of unrest describe it to me to know the feelings ... what do you feel? How does your body feel? What is it doing?

*GIULIA*: *I can't feel it now*

*TERAPEUTA*: You can start moving your body without feeling much, then it's the body moving, so if you were nervous and turned around, do it here so you'll see that the body itself will evoke the situation.

> Giulia starts moving and talking in a low voice

*GIULIA*: *Here, now I just have to sleep, I am uncomfortable, shit, I have to put on earplugs, what a bother*

> She continues expressing her unrest, grumbles, moves. I encourage her and tell her to go on, obviously I talk in a low voice but not too much, so the rest of the group can hear, then I ask her what this agitation means.

*GIULIA*: *I am afraid, afraid that someone, that he touches me ...*

*TERAPEUTA*: Now go back in time and feel this fear of being invaded, as you felt it as a child, but keep that restless feeling

I always start from what the person brings to the session but then I look for similar situations in the past. I do it also because I know that with her partner nothing until now justifies her agitation. She keeps moving and jerking, turning around in her bed. She keeps her eyes closed, grumbles and stretches her legs:

GIULIA: *Ah, yes, I remember when I was a child in my cot I did not want them to read me fairy tales, I was afraid of them, but I liked to hold mummy's hand*

TERAPEUTA: OK, go back to that important moment and go back there holding mummy's hand

GIULIA: *It's lovely!*

TERAPEUTA: Be a child again and feel the warmth of this hand but hear also mummy reading these scary tales, go back to the moment where there is pleasure for the hand and fear of the tale. How old are you?

GIULIA: *I'm four*

TERAPEUTA: You are four and you hold mummy's hand, what do you feel?

GIULIA: *It's lovely ... I feel ... like shivers*

TERAPEUTA: What tales is she reading?

GIULIA: *Sleeping beauty and I was afraid ... I was terrorized when the witch told her, "One day you'll prick your finger and you'll die"*

I signal to a group member to come closer, take Giulia's hand and then tell Sleeping beauty, she starts in a soft warm voice. I choose a person that is also a mother, she is sweet and warm. Before inviting her to come closer I asked her silently if she was willing and she nodded in assent. In this group all members are willing to help others reconstruct their past situations. To have persons available to act the parts in a proper way is indispensable for using these techniques.

TERAPEUTA: (after a while) What do you feel, Giulia?

GIULIA: *At the beginning I don't care if I am afraid ... it's odd, I like that she holds my hand but then I am afraid of what can happen ... I am always afraid of the future, of what will happen, it's like I had at the same time the safety of the hand and the fear of growing up.*

TERAPEUTA: Stay a little longer in touch with this fear. What did you do then with your mother? Was there something you could do to stop her or could you ask her to do something else? What would you like to do now?

GIULIA:        *Mummy, can you tell a different story?*
TERAPEUTA:     More, can you ask for more, maybe she changes tale but everything remains as it was. Is there anything else you can tell her?

> I am insisting because Giulia already has permission to ask for what she wants but I think she is just asking for concrete behaviors, as she already learned to do with her partner. I think here she lacks a more comprehensive request, she needs to be reassured, but she also needs a tighter relation with her mother. At this point I know she was not protected as a child, but I don't know what she will say. She has always had to be *Strong* and give up being a child, she has always done everything by herself in order not to make her very anxious mother worry. She told me that when she was about six she had packed a couple of things in a bundle and had fled home. She obviously got lost a couple of blocks from home and was found. But this story made me understand how she felt in her family and how already age six she already felt she could do all by herself.

GIULIA:        *Mummy I am afraid of evil persons, I am afraid of death, that you die and I don't want to hear these tales.*
TERAPEUTA:     What do you want from your mother that you never asked her?
GIULIA:        *I would like to stay close to her ...*

> This is the turning point. She always tried to run away from her mother but had remained home with her even when she could have moved in with her partner a few years ago. She felt a very strong link, she told me, but quite contradictory. Even if they were always in conflict, she had become a true *Rescuer* for her mother, she felt the need to reassure her mother all the time that her initial efforts at autonomy would not lead to the catastrophes her anxious mother always prophesized. Even after she had finally been able, during treatment, to go and live on her own, their link was still very strong. Giulia spent hours on the phone almost every day telling her mother that she was fine, to calm her and tell her everything went well also workwise, even if it was not totally true. To recognize now the need to have her mother close to her and to be able to say it so openly in

front of everybody was a relevant recognition of how she had missed a healthy closeness with proper roles, where a mother is a mother and a daughter a daughter and not the opposite as it had been in the past. Only by accepting the persistence of her need for protection and the original love drive toward her mother Giulia will be able to change her relation to her mother and to others.

TERAPEUTA: Tell her directly

GIULIA: *Mummy, I want to come in your bed, I want to stay with you ... I am afraid!*

TERAPEUTA: What would you like your mother to answer you?

GIULIA: (starting to cry) *It's OK, all will be well, you don't need to worry about everything, life is scary, I have to go on even when I feel something is wrong.*

The group member reassures her with maternal gestures, then when I invite her to do so, she gets closer and Giulia, crying, hugs her and clings to her, she lets herself go with a happy expression. This is finally the expression of Giulia's need for reassurance from her mother and at the same time an explosion of filial love that she had never been able to express because she was too busy running away and defending herself from her mother. At the beginning the other group member just showed her willingness to be available because it was Giulia who needed to feel the drive to become active and hug. Group members have learned that they must never substitute the other and facilitate their activation too much. It's Giulia who must change and for her the change is to take the initiative and hug and be hugged, to let herself be truly protected. She is the one who needs to learn how to be protected and to feel finally a child who can ask. As we know, Giulia needed always to run away from this mother who scared her with her tragic forebodings. I leave them there in silence for a while, we are all moved, then without any intervention from me, Giulia releases the hug, sits up and opens her eyes. We all smile.

TERAPEUTA: We have to learn to distinguish what you perceived as a good mother from the other, let's call her the bad, anxious mother. You have to get in contact with the good mother, the one who gave you this wonderful body, this liveliness, this cleverness and on the other side scared you to death. For too long you have forgotten the good mother that was close to you and told you fairy tales while you were too busy keeping away that anxious, controlling mother full of fears who was so scared and passed on to you insecurity about yourself and life. In your infantile world only the scared mother could prevail, the one you internalized, but there was the other too and from now on before falling asleep, if you still feel restless, remember your mother's fears, maybe she tried to exorcize them with the fairy tales, maybe she thought she was protecting you. You can ask your partner to be patient and understanding with you and you can tell yourself that you still need protection. Scared children can be comforted but they need to be able to ask the right persons. Your partner seems to be the right person, your child part has chosen the right person, now you can ask him and in a short time you too will be able to relax.

Giulia and the other group member now sit next to each other and hold hands, they listen and stroke each other tenderly, this is the crystallization phase, the rational view, understanding mother's limitations but also her good intentions. No one can think that she scared that child so much if not to protect her. She certainly intended for her daughter to lead a better life than hers. She was warning her without realizing that in that way she was creating useless fears and a feeling of fragility.

TERAPEUTA:  (addressing the whole group): What a nice example this mother: on one side she holds her daughter's hand and on the other she tells terrifying stories and you can do nothing because you are scared and if you ask her to stop she could leave, so you cannot say what you wish.
You were already a child scared by her anxiety and were always alarmed.
We must disactivate this alarm and the best way to do it in treatment is to consider that that alarm was understandable, healthy, you were truly scared, what was unhealthy was to keep the alarm and not be able to say "*Mummy, stop telling me those stories, otherwise how can I sleep?*"
It's like someone suddenly waking you when you are sleeping. You have always lived in this climate and inside you resided an alarm you couldn't turn off because it was caused

by the same person that should have protected your Child part.

Then your mother has always been anxious so you have to realize that your fears ... were hers and she passed them on to you because of the unfortunate life she had had as a child.

GIULIA:   *Yes, it's true, now I remember, I had forgotten, she has always been afraid of the dark, even as a grownup, even now!*

TERAPEUTA:   Then you know what you could do? You can go see your mum and tell her a tale, the nicest you know, with a happy ending ... and you thank her for how she tried to protect you, even if she herself was not at ease. Your risk is that you do the same with Tobia, first you put him in the role of the good mother but then you feel restless and you make him become the bad mother.

GIULIA:   *You are right, that's how I do, from a certain moment on he seems unable to do the things I want, while I am the one forgetting the earplugs, going to bed too late, in a bed that is too small. I am the one unable to take care of herself.*

TERAPEUTA:   You project onto Tobia the image of the bad mother that did not comfort you enough.

You know how best to sleep, what are the ideal conditions, suggest them to Tobia, let him help you but do not delegate to him how, you are the one who needs to learn how to protect herself. Your mother was always worried and scared for what had actually happened to her, in her life, but nothing of that happened to you, so you should remember that your life is a lot better than hers.

One more thing. Restlessness is always an obstacle to doing things, yours was hugging your mother to find comfort and love her and maybe also to make her stop. When you are restless today it means that you cannot take the next step that is go and hug or go and tell what you want from others.

You have to be active to get what you want.

Restlessness makes you passive or better you are restless because you are blocking the loving urge to go and ask. You feel you want it but you deny it, your movements are useless, a coming and going even with your body where energy is never exhausted because it cannot reach its end, that is, to satisfy the true urge: "Mummy, I need you to protect me, I need you".

A GROUP MEMBER *asks*: *But fairy tales, even the scary ones, aren't they useful?*

TERAPEUTA:   They are, but only if mother is protective and the child is relaxed, then they make the child feel safe in their mother's arms in front of dangers. This is their function. They scare you a little but in a protective environment, they help you grow as a positive Parent by introjecting the protective power of a mother, but when mother is anxious with the fairy tale she re-creates a dangerous world that she cannot defeat. If the environment does not protect, these tales are forever scary.

> Giulia came back triumphant at the next meeting, she slept longer than usual during the week, with or without Tobia. Then they decided to buy a double bed for his flat because when she stayed the night they slept in two single beds or squeezed in one of them and he had to wait for her to fall asleep, cuddling her, then he could go to sleep too. She never dared ask him to buy a double bed but then she nagged him because he wasn't welcoming enough. A nice *psychological trick*: from victim she turned into persecutor of her partner who was never protective/RESCUER enough. Giulia also went to see her mother, told her she loves her and asked for advice, she really wanted to see how it would end. But her mother asked her, "*You ask me for advice? You always told me not to worry, that you knew how to do everything. Come on, you are a grown woman now, what do you want me to know, ask Tobia instead!*". Giulia was almost fainting. When we really change it happens that others too change. It is not our goal to change persons that are not in treatment but it happens often that when an attitude changes, especially when it is with one's parents or with one's partner, a virtuous energy circle is activated that introduces new relational possibilities. This is what Giulia wrote to me two years after the end of her treatment. I quote this letter because I want to stress that even without working directly on her body we succeeded in recovering a healthy and energetic physicality thus holistically relaxing the whole system.
>
> Maybe where we start from is not so important.

*At the end of an intense day of work I am thinking of you, like many other nights when I imagine letters that then I don't write. What is happening? It happens that blooming continues, I feel that I am in the place I wanted to be. On September 20 I completed the master course, which means to start a route for becoming good. I am no longer anxious.*

*I know where I am, what I know, how to do it, what I need to learn to become good.*

*So if I take things well I am glad, if I do something wrong or if there's something I don't know how to do, I try to find the best solution and I stopped criticizing myself.*

*I no longer feel obliged to study for duty but I am doing it for pleasure.*

*But most of all, a lot of energy that was locked inside me is now free and needs to find a form because at the moment I am still too busy with work but I know it will be better later on.*

*For about two years I haven't had a pain anywhere in my body, my back and knees are fine, I practice a lot of sports that I introduced gradually and are now my main activities. I really feel like moving, recovering all the lost sensations, all that I had left aside with my obsession of having to study: running, swimming, climbing (for what I can, don't imagine things).*

*Today for fun a patient made me try to dance and I felt the same feeling I had years ago when I was in an intensive group and I danced with Mario.*

*So I called him and I think one of the next forms of my enthusiasm will be dancing, for what I can. Another great success is my relation to my mother, no more fights and anger and we even recovered some tenderness and cuddles.*

*This year she hesitatingly asked me and I rented a place at the seaside for her in September (my parents never went on holiday and my mother has anxiety fits only thinking of traveling, for her Romagna is the same as Patagonia for me).*

*Knew that either they would not go or they would not like anything, but in March I had already organized everything and as soon as she arrived there she started texting very sweet thanks (like "I feel like a child that the parents send for the first time to summer camp, thanks Giulia, I taught you how to walk, you how to sail").*

*She read Garcia Marquez on the beach instead of St. Augustine or the Bible, she picked tons of ugly stones thinking they were beautiful. I went to see them over the weekend to check how they were and we were all very well…"*

## Second example: Tommaso

Tommaso is 40 and has been in treatment for six years with interruptions because he spent long periods abroad for work.

Now he is back in Italy and a couple of years ago was finally able to join a group and his attendance is constant.

He has very low self-esteem, he is so Pleasing that he almost lost his personality. When he started treatment he was cyclically depressed, did not get out of his home for weeks, kept the blinds down and alternated periods of isolation with phases in which he frantically looked for approval, he was often besieged by bouts of anxiety that led him to work manically, looking for perfection in anything he did to avoid any criticism or mistake.

He had a symbiotic romantic relation with a girl, they were a mutual safety line for each other but it was him who was always available and, in order to try to be loved, he was totally and subserviently devoted to her.

At the time of this session Tommaso had left her when he had realized that he was too dependent on that relation that was too limiting, so with great guilt but with the support of the group he had decided to try some new different relations and had managed to give value to his autonomy also in love matters.

His mother was a very distressed person, for some periods under drug treatment, had divorced his father when Tommaso was a child and had poured onto him all her suffocating love and aggression. She often beat him up when she experienced anger attacks that her son tried to sedate with love.

He had never felt important for or valued by her and although he was rather controlled and devalued, he had never been able to separate or rebel. He considered his depression and performance anxiety his own fault; he was never right, good, mature enough.

His father was totally nonexistent, and he remembered only occasional games and some failed effort at getting closer when he was an adult.

Once he left that couple relation that he considered a gilded retreat/jail, he was now facing his difficulty in managing his own life trying to understand what he really liked in a woman.

In this period his Natural Child, creative, enthusiastic, warm, full of initiatives was also, after many years of uncertainty and fear, finally free to express himself, since he had left his girlfriend the autonomy drive was starting to move inside him.

But he was unable to protect himself and make choices directed to a stable and economically viable future.

TOMMASO:     *I want to dedicate myself to me, I am tired of living with this*
             *performance anxiety, I feel I am going backwards because I*
             *can't work like I would like. The jobs I got this year I accepted*
             *them lightly, I felt like doing but now I have to prepare an activ-*
             *ity for a group pf 30 persons and it all seems very heavy. I would*
             *like to free myself from this feeling even though from an organi-*
             *zational point of view I think I am fine now with this task.*
TERAPEUTA:   So you are not going backwards.

             I never let these devaluations unattended (*I feel I am*
             *going backwards*), in particular with a formerly depressed
             person even if, like in this case, after this brief mention I
             prefer to move on and touch more relevant aspects.

TOMMASO:     *Then why do I feel so bad that I almost did not come here*
             *because of the anxiety caused by this job?*

*TERAPEUTA*: Something is lacking, if you are already organized you are doing something you didn't do earlier, it's already good. If there's something lacking that prevents you from being relaxed, don't forget you are already doing things different from before, you told me you were well organized, it is fine, isn't it?

*TOMMASO*: *I realized that I am doing it, that the way I am doing this last job is different, I gathered more information, I discussed my salary and times of payment.*

*TERAPEUTA*: OK, let's take a mattress. (I make him lie on it and tell him) Do you see how you boycott yourself, you don't miss the chance to berate yourself saying you are going backwards! But let's forget that now, close your eyes and say everything that comes to your mind thinking you have a job to do, speak freely, imagine no one is listening.

> He usually talks a lot, he runs after his thoughts, he risks, and I with him, to jump from one matter to another, so I lead him immediately to a mildly regressive condition to put him in contact with his emotions and fears as fast as possible; his rationalizations are a trap.

*TOMMASO*: *Even just lying here makes me think a lot, I think that my loneliness in this thing weighs heavily, I think that I have to manage all by myself from the creative to the organizational part.*

> "Here we are: I think a lot ..." He is very often lost in thought.

*TERAPEUTA*: OK, go on, I feel alone, I know I am alone ...

*TOMMASO*: *I am afraid, I am scared and this feeling of fear was very strong in the past days, when there's a lot of time before completing a job it is the most difficult moment for me but when I am there working and seeing the finishing line I can relax and anxiety leaves, but before it was pretty high.*

> Here he opens his eyes, sits up looking for a pillow but doesn't ask me for it, and finds one.

*TERAPEUTA*: This is already relevant, what just happened, while I ask you to let go and to say all that comes to your mind, you immediately need to sit up, open your eyes, you don't tell me you are uncomfortable, you go your own way. I consider your sitting up like a way to put yourself on watch.

> The choice whether to stress his change of state or his effort at going back to thoughts rather than stay on emotions is usually quite difficult. Should I stress it? Should I tell him? Do I provide some early conclusion? Am I too meticulous and obsessive? Should I just drop it? In any case the observation should concern an issue consistent with what he is doing so that we can tackle it more directly, not to move the attention elsewhere. In afterthought, it was a good choice to intervene because he gets the observation immediately.

TOMMASO: *Here's another thing you just mentioned: on watch, it's as if I was always on watch, any thought and action I am on watch, if I am doing well, if I am doing right or if I am making decisions in time, I put myself on watch and this makes me dizzy, just like now.*

TERAPEUTA: Stay there, on the feeling ... what do you mean by dizzy? What do you feel?

TOMMASO: *It's voices coming in all the time.*

TERAPEUTA: What voices?

TOMMASO: *The call to attention, to being vigilant.*

TERAPEUTA: Let's use them; you try to be these voices and talk to Tommaso, how can these voices put him on watch, what do they say? Interpret them, be a voice.

TOMMASO: *It's a constant buzz.*

TERAPEUTA: Be the buzz, let me hear it, add some words.

TOMMASO: *Mm, you are late ... mmm always doing new difficult things, you can't do it, you are late ... then there are good words that say: try not to think about it, ii doesn't matter, take your time, enjoy the rest too, you're good.*

TERAPEUTA: Go back to the initial buzzing voices.

TOMMASO: *You are alone, you are taking a leap in the void.*

TERAPEUTA: Go deeper, take a leap in the void, what does this particular sentence mean, how does it fit in your life – take a leap in the void.

TOMMASO: *The feeling I have is anxiety all around and there's a void around, I feel the lack of a boundary, of solid ground.*

TERAPEUTA: Stay on the feeling of lack of boundaries, of solid ground and void around you and go even deeper and back in time, try and feel the most ancient feeling you feel when you think of a void without solid ground around you, without boundaries and it's a very physical sensation.

TOMMASO:    *I don't have a hand that makes me feel present and alive, capable of living, as if it was the proof that I exist.*

> He now talks very slowly; I understand he is feeling in the depth that something ancient is emerging. I know what he lacked: his mother gave him no boundaries, even as a child he was in his room and his mother never let him close the door, in part to control him but mostly, as we learned later, because she didn't want to be alone. She was the one who wanted his company, he took care of her, he made over for the lack of a partner and this is what he did with all his girlfriends, a great RESCUER already as a child, always worried for the others.

TERAPEUTA:    Say this thing: I need boundaries to live!
TOMMASO:    *Yes, definitely ... I need boundaries to exist.*
TERAPEUTA:    It's a very old thing, you are afraid of being alone and feel a void around you, you need a hand to give you a boundary that helps you to exist, you feel the emotion inside you ... try to ask.
TOMMASO:    *How can you ask existence to someone other than you?*
TERAPEUTA:    It is possible to ask for a boundary, a limit, a support. This you can ask.
TOMMASO:    *I feel like asking for a hand but it is not the hand and I have always wondered, it is not the hand I need, it is not help, the hand comforts me but it is not the hand that comforts me. It's absurd!*

> This is typical of him. When a need emerges he immediately thinks about it to see if he can ask himself, or better his first question is if he is allowed to feel that need. So I bring him back to the point that is to express what he always lacked, his true need.

TERAPEUTA:    What do you need, of what can't you do without?
TOMMASO:    *Support.*
TERAPEUTA:    You feel the loneliness one feels when there is no support.

> He starts crying. It doesn't happen often, in general in the latest period he was rather assertive when he intervened during treatment, emotions of this kind had not emerged in him for a long time.

TOMMASO:        *... I am lost and I start confusing everything, all my thoughts are confused.*

TERAPEUTA:    It's better now, now don't think, just feel, feel that you are alone and without support, without a limit and a boundary that gives a limit to your existence, where you are and where is the rest of the world, if you let yourself be invaded by this feeling you will then feel what you need, what you are lacking, now here.

> I try to go deeper in his feelings. I know he has been taking care of his anxious mother from very early on. She was often treated with drugs and psychotherapy, I know he always took care of her and was very scared by her panic and anxiety attacks.

TOMMASO:        *I am lacking the serenity of knowing that I am not going to die, that nothing happens, that I am not making a dreadful mess.*

TERAPEUTA:    You are doing well now, you are in it, you are in your needs and you are asking for something you have done without all your life long and it's a boundary, I can do until that point and it's fine, when you ask for a hand this is what you want – to the point where I exist, to the point I can reach with work – you said earlier I feel alone, I am afraid, I need a hand, these are the words, the thoughts and fears you had as a child. I ask you to repeat the request for a hand, since you feel alone and are afraid, you need to feel where your limit is, you can live now your solitude.

TOMMASO (crying):    *It's as if I didn't want to feel totally the pain for what I am lacking and I didn't want to realize that I am truly alone and however nothing happens, I am here and alive, even if I am alone.*

TERAPEUTA:    That's right, good, this is what you are discovering that you are alive even if alone and that the presence of another person is not salvation, is not indispensable, but it could help you to be able to count on someone and maybe today someone is there.

> I touch him lightly on the shoulder to make him feel my presence and he is even more moved but the rest he has to do by himself. This is a very difficult passage, I know his mother did not allow him to have a boundary, or better she invaded him constantly, I know that not even his father had set a boundary, on the contrary, he left him alone with a distressed and disturbed mother. I want to support the feeling of lack, that was quite real

and still is, to give him the permission to let himself be helped and at the same time receive a physical support, just as real in the present to make him feel that it is possible not to do everything alone. In the present I am here and the group is here to support this child that has to learn to let others help him, has to learn to ask for the help he could not ask to his parents. But he must not receive closeness through a compliant and servile availability, rather through asking for what he needs. He has to do it by himself but then ask for help only for what is necessary. All these are corrective emotional experiences and at the same time are a way for learning a gesture that was missing at the time. The goal is developing self-protection and the autonomy drive.

TOMMASO:      *... I want to put this thing inside me, I do.*
TERAPEUTA:   Yes, put it inside,
TOMMASO:      *... I keep looking for it outside even if I will never find it.*
TERAPEUTA:   You are right there, how can you find it outside if you don't feel it here, the void was outside you, not inside, the void was your mother's inability to protect you and your father's absence, the void you felt was their absence, their inability to give you support and leaving to you the choice of limits. You have lived without this convinced that your insecurity was your fault.
TOMMASO:      *... put the void inside me.*
TERAPEUTA:   Exactly, now you have to put inside something else instead of that void, is there anything that can substitute your mother, that gives you a sense of where you end and you can't go beyond. You don't know how to give yourself a limit because she did not give it to you. Did she ever tell you: stop my son, this is good.
TOMMASO:      *... what I remember is how she hit me when I asked for something and insisted too much.*
TERAPEUTA:   When she couldn't stand it any longer she hit you so you discovered that you existed, today you have to give yourself the limit stopping to hit yourself, stopping to criticize yourself and accepting that you are doing your best and this is already enough to know you are good.
TOMMASO:      *... I am afraid of what will come next ... because I don't know if I'll make it.*
TERAPEUTA:   This happens only when you have exaggerated goals. In that case you don't know if you'll make it, but if you set the limit for yourself, then you know you can do it, if you look for

perfection you will always be afraid of not reaching it, that's obvious, but if you give yourself a reachable limit, you set it. This is why it is hard for you to go to bed at peace, you can never say "today I have done enough, it's OK to stop here!" Not everything needs to be perfect, you are good at your work but you have to accept that you set a limit, not exhaustion, anxiety or blows.

TOMMASO:     *... But the others judge me.*

TERAPEUTA:   No, here you are the one to judge because the others always expect less than what you give, we have always known this, the others accept you as you are, you set the limit, relax, you don't need to do more than what you normally do, try to understand, a mother that is never happy with you, that never tells you to stop, that doesn't set limits and the son goes on and on and then blows come to close the action.

TOMMASO:     *... I want to do things with calm, I don't like to do them badly.*

He is coming back to today, he is starting to think again but I want him to finish the old action that he had not been able to finish with his mother also physically with his body, so I think I need to make him have a corrective experience on the impossibility of the past, which was not a prohibition, given the situation, but a real impossibility, how could he ask his mother for help? I tell this sentence slowly.

TERAPEUTA:   Very well, but you have to set a limit to yourself and be able to say OK for today I have done enough. I am the one who decides.

TOMMASO:     *... I am not good at this.*

TERAPEUTA:   You know that the lack of a limit is something that happened in reality and that to obtain a limit at the end of an action you have to receive blows to be able to say "yes, she noticed me". In order for the others to notice you don't need to harm yourself and get dead tired, you exist from now on independently from others, now stay still with my hand on your shoulder, feel my closeness, listen to what we have done until now, feel what you need, feel it physically and emotionally with your body.

He doesn't move or talk for a while, all the others are silent and that gesture starts becoming more and more meaningful, then he takes my hand that was still on his shoulder, squeezes it and brings it to his heart. This is the first step. He can feel that he needs help but also he can feel how to separate and decide the duration of closeness. This new closeness cannot be totalizing and unconditional as in childhood.

TERAPEUTA:   Yes, keep my hand there but you know that sooner or later you'll have to let go, you decide when and then let it go.

He cries a little and squeezes my hand then slowly after a while he lifts it from his shoulder and lets go. I wait for a while to see if he wants something else, then I get up and return to my chair.

TOMMASO:   ... *It was great* (he gets up and takes his seat again).
TERAPEUTA:   Is there anything else to say? Shall we stop here?
TOMMASO:   *Yes it's enough, I got it.*
TERAPEUTA:   (addressing all) I only want to add, Tommaso, that this problem of your boundaries was created very early on, that's why it was so invasive in many aspects of your life. Think of your relationship with women, how you always let yourself be invaded by their needs, how it was always hard for you to say enough! to them too, to say where you could reach and were willing to be available: up to here it's ok for me too, beyond this, no.
It is the same, as we have seen, at work, the limit you can give yourself now is your evaluation of how tired you are, of the steps you planned to reach the goal. You have to decide that taking into account also your other projects, you need to learn how to plan.
In this you can and should ask someone for help but without confusing yourself with their needs, as you did with you mum. If you are the one asking, you are also the one defining the help you request.
"I need this much, nothing more".
Enough with being immersed totally in your work and in your relations, enough with exhaustion to be able to stop, you have to be able to go to bed at night with an internal Parent that tells you,
dear Tommaso, now it's enough, it's more than enough. OK?
Or better, plan your times of work and leisure beforehand with enough flexibility, then manage the situations and go where you want.
TOMMASO:   *... It sounds like a dream!*
TERAPEUTA:   Definitely and you know that dreams come true, don't you?

They all laugh.

> Tommaso has started organizing his life according to a plan, every once in a while he still makes some mistake but he has become perfectly autonomous, sometimes exaggerating, sometimes finding himself confused again but he has to learn how to do it. To become autonomous requires a constant training. On the other hand he is a freelance worker and often worked with people who became "friends". He always risked to confuse the areas and let himself be caught too much as he trusted the other's total availability. In time some painful experiences have helped him become even more capable of choosing the distance and putting himself at the center of his life.
>
> I accepted and welcomed in different ways his phone calls and requests of individual sessions. At times he called me at the last minute expecting a total availability on my part. If I could I obviously obliged, but often I refused. I wanted to be the person that although willing to help him was not always unconditionally there. The same happened in his love life; after his first symbiotic and very long relationship for a while he avoided romantic relations, he needed to find the right distance and his own centrality with women. For what I know after the end of his treatment he found both: he has married and has a daughter. He definitely has become a man.

It really seems quite evident to me, in closing this chapter, that corrective experiences can be deeper and more definitive when they are experienced both emotionally and physically, closing an experience that was fixed in the negative behaviors of many years past.

In all the cases I mentioned, as is evident from a certain moment on, the actual need for protection and containment was not only unmet but inhibited, hampered and badly managed.

For this reason the natural propensities (in the first case survival and love and in the second autonomy) and the related abilities not only could not be expressed properly but also lost their power.

In situations like these the (also loving) relation between therapist and patient can help because for many it is with the therapist that the process of reparation can be implemented at last.

This is why Orbecchi (2015) wrote:

> Without the therapist's capacity to provide an empathic response to the patient's attachment need there is no possibility of recovering in the other that self-esteem that is the basis from which one can find the external and internal safety for exploring and building the meaning of one's life.

To return with the mind to the experiences of the past allows to:

• Give permission to express the healthy drives that had lost power and develop the related abilities (such as asking for help, hugging, wishing, exploring, etc.)

- Let the original needs emerge (stimulus, recognition, structure)
- Provide an adequate parental response in the here and now
- Make the patient responsible for acting differently from now on

I don't know if I conveyed in these past two chapters the climate created in groups by these therapeutic activities, but I hope that readers can have a glimpse of the deep feelings and closeness that these activities elicit in all the persons present.

They feel they are reliving the same situations in which they had tried in the past to express their natural orientation.

The Child parts that were upset, lost, disappointed, scared, relive those moments as soon as they access these regressive conditions.

For all those present it is like watching a child that is starting to walk. While you watch them moving in space toward arms open to take them in, they smile full of hope even if they are at the same time afraid and uncertain for the previous falls and failures. But when finally they wobbling reach their goal and collapse in those open arms, we all clap our hands and celebrate because in that precise moment we know immediately that something touching and awesome has just happened.

Something that for all of us has been an extraordinary passage.

All, some more and some less, have gone through those awkward moments to obtain the basic Permissions for survival, all have in their memory a drive that tries to realize and a family that responds, more or less, a thousand times to that drive.

To be able to love one's mother and father, to be able to trust and rely, to be able to ask for help and feel supported, to be able to express one's attachment and feel safe, to be able to look at the world with love and joy are infantile experiences crucial for all and at the same time impressive.

They remain because they are basic messages for the realization of our humanity, embedded in the most archaic memory both when the outcome was positive and then it was dramatic.

I think that to relive those moments cannot but elicit deep feelings and true joy in groups and can make all the members resonate together enhancing indelibly a common brotherhood. We all have been and are like this.

We want to live and love.

## Bibliography

Karpman S. (1968) Fairy tales and script drama analysis. In *Transactional Anayisis Bulletin*, 7(26): 39–43.

Orbecchi M. (2015) *Biologia dell'anima. Teoria dell'evoluzione e psicoterapia.* (*Biology of the Soul. Evolutionary Theory and Psychotherapy*). Torino, Bollati Boringhieri.

# Chapter 12

# Nourishes joy the pain

Emotional life is certainly a relevant feature of groups.

It is probably the most remarkable element that makes them different from individual therapy. In evening groups, in the longer ones and most of all in the residential ones lasting two or three days, patients are so engrossed that they let their emotions emerge more easily.

Feeling, first of all, and then expressing one's emotions is one of the most important abilities of human beings (I think it is not necessary to stress it again, suffice to read any of Damasio's books [1994, 1999, 2021]). Basic emotions that cause distress (anger, fear, sadness, and the feelings related to them) inform us that something is wrong in our existence and therefore they are indispensable alarms for survival, while other emotions that elicit wellbeing (joy and in general all positive feelings) inform us that something good and favorable happened, and they are the nourishment and reward of our actions.

All these concepts have already been illustrated in the previous chapters.

What I want to stress here is how emotions are often sedated or deviated in childhood.

In all families there are allowed emotions and prohibited emotions, but sometimes the whole system made of feeling/manifesting/learning from experience is undermined, a system that is what we need in life to understand what is going on and therefore to decide whether to change or confirm our behavior.

If a child is prevented for a long time or violently from expressing their drives (and this means to go well beyond containment, that is however necessary and healthy for a child), their defensive response cannot but be pervaded with anger, fear or sadness and later evidenced by the related behaviors of aggression, restlessness, and withdrawal.

These responses will be followed by further parental responses in an escalation of confrontations and misunderstandings that will self-feed and where usually the most dependent and fragile will lose.

Although it is not always the child to be the most fragile.

Parents usually do their best to sedate these manifestations of dissent, they try to convince their children that all is well, that they are not allowed to feel what they feel, they often associate different insults and definitions to those

DOI: 10.4324/9781003303831-12

emotions, in an effort at making them more understandable and acceptable. They say their child is tired, lazy, rebellious, uncontrollable, moody, thus redefining and distorting the child's initial propensities and their emotional responses to the frustrations received. So the child will feel rejected and helpless twice.

The first time because their propensities have not been welcomed as they would have liked and the second because they could not even express the ensuing suffering.

The result is that often adult persons that start a treatment, although showing quite relevant problems, tend to minimize them, describe them with emotional detachment and consider them contingent phenomena that have nothing to do with their history because they were taught to see them in this way.

The causes are buried deep in their unconscious or, if you prefer, in their implicit memory.

They are distressed for the consequences of their present behaviors, not for their frustrated nature, not for their held-back propensities, not for the deviated course of their structural growth. They bring their discomfort for what is taking place in the present but they tell themselves a story of the world that is complete and comprehensive, well-structured and, something even more serious, they believe in it.

A Script is an old narrative that includes the therapist too, at least at the beginning, and if the patients realize that they need to change, they tend to do it by changing as little as possible their representation of themselves and of their existence.

Usually they are totally unaware of this and therefore they ask us to help them to stop being distressed and overcome their problem without opening old graves or discovering skeletons in their closets.

I think this is the reason why in the past few years the psychotherapies focused only on the "here and now" received great approval.

A relevant part of psychoanalyses has often enhanced the fear of reflecting on the past with an attitude similar to that of a sadistic speleologist who does not look for treasures of lost humanity but for monsters to kill.

Common sense still sees psychotherapists as "seekers of souls" to quote the old and beautiful book by Groddeck (1919), hunting for invented traumas, manic defenses, perverse and distorted sexuality, shadows and ghosts, penis envy, death instinct. In the original book cover of 1921, as a "funny" example, we see a psychoanalyst studying the pubis of a girl with a magnifying glass! Down there, in the unconscious, they thought there must be something rotten, uncontrolled sexuality, antisocial primitive impulses, suppressed aggression, the death instinct as an original sin to be cleansed, not the wonders of our natural state.

The widely feared "removed" Is instead often an unexpressed original distress that can at times be also aggressive because those that we tend to show as adults are usually the emotions and behaviors that we were allowed to show, not the genuine ones related to the events happened.

These are substitute and "parasite" emotions and stereotyped behaviors that later emerge, independent of their natural and original function. Fear is often hidden under embarrassment, sadness under shame, anger toward the others is turned against oneself in self-harming behaviors or becomes anger and destructive aggression.

At times emotional life is dulled by a permanent damper; at others, causing the most serious cases, is definitively muted with outcomes like narcissism, alexithymia, psychopathy.

So one is spared the anxiety due to abandonment but becomes isolated and passive and retreats more and more from the possibility of obtaining the warm closeness that had been denied at the beginning of life.

And this is the most unhappy and paradoxical negative side of our Scripts: we will continue to disown our basic drives and to choose behaviors and opinions on ourselves and the world that will take us ever further from the possibility to realize our nature.

We become our own jailers.

Healthy functioning is often confused or compromised; patients no longer understand the origin of their distress or they interpret it in the wrong way because the emotional signals they have been allowed to use are different from the original authentic ones.

More and more patients come to our consulting rooms pervaded by a comprehensive pseudo-rationality; they understand that something is wrong, maybe because they have some psychosomatic symptoms (typical of persons that cannot feel much) or because their third marriage ended badly.

They are so "emotionally anesthetized" that they talk about their failures with a terrifying detachment, as if they did not concern them at all, as if their need for love did not exist.

Then, almost always, slowly, truth emerges.

An empathic, patient, and welcoming listening can help them access the deeper levels of their experience and at last tears flow.

And they are always the tears of a very young child that had to stop crying or protesting in front of a mother or father who started by frustrating them and ended up not allowing them to be sad or angry.

We often say, ironically, that one goes to treatment to pay for crying and often it is true; what never happens, instead, is that crying, when it is finally related to what actually caused that sadness, becomes an open door to a forgotten "Script room" (Karpman, 1968, Cosso, 2013), it sheds light on a scene that has been totally hidden in the darkness of the past.

And it always shows great truths.

For me it is difficult to describe that feeling, it's as if a mother came back to retrieve a child that had been abandoned for years in an orphanage. At that moment parent and child recognize each other and the little one can run into her arms to tell her all that happened: vexations, solitude, boredom, and more and they know they will find acceptance, understanding, and protection.

One in the arms of the other with tears melting all defenses, they are able to recover the thread that had bound indissolubly their lives at birth.

What seemed Impossible to express to their parents then is now accepted and recognized as true suffering by the therapist, by the group and by the patients themselves.

In those moments, in front of the Child part that spills the beans the Parent Ego State is activated, and it hugs with feeling and compassion. It is the intra-psychic meeting of parts of the self, of the suffering Natural Child and their Parent finally welcoming and comforting.

It is truth coming to the surface in the patient's intrapsychic life, the various parts of personality recognize, accept, integrate, love each other in the end. And inner peace is established.

It is the same also if we need to express anger: a scream always denied that can finally come out from the depth to shout "Enough! Stop it! No! Go away!" or "Help! Someone do something, I am scared! Mummy!"

Whatever was the past suffering, it must be now accepted and understood so that it can receive a proper response that frees the interrupted evolution and introduces new pathways of experience and alternative adequate behaviors in the mind.

The denied emotions are always fear, pain, and anger, the deepest and most ancient that all human beings feel when they are abused, abandoned, treated with indifference, reified, assaulted, and when their natural drives have been crushed.

The earlier the inhibitions set in, the greater the damage they cause, which means that we have to reach the earliest emotions to free the persons and let them express themselves to create an information channel that leads to different behaviors from the ones they learned at the beginning of their lives, to restrained capacities, to forgotten experiences, to the "natural precursors" that need to be reactivated.

It's like going back in the past and reopening a dam that by preventing the river water to flow made the surrounding countryside barren.

The masks and false selves, character structures, adaptations, whatever names different psychological schools use for "protections/defenses", are always a difficult obstacle to overcome to reach the underlying actual pain and the condition that determined it.

But when we reach the point of treatment when we are able to remove them, we free voices that are so beautiful that all members of the group welcome them with joy and satisfaction, as if they were seeing the labor of a difficult childbirth that is finally accomplished: the return to a natural life.

However, despite what many of those who rely on emotional catharsis think, therapeutic work does not end here.

Given how our mind works, we have awoken only one alternative possibility for life, we opened a door and let energy flow out, we recovered a drive and saw alternative behaviors, a crucial step, inevitable in my opinion, but this change is *not* yet complete and definitive.

In time our mental habits always return. If that new road is not trodden constantly, rewarded by joy, and supported by constant encouragement, it risks to return to being unknown and impassable.

Everything will go back to its previous state with the additional burden of a sense of failure, inability, mistrust, resignation, that will hamper all further efforts at changing.

As I summarized in the table concerning the phases of therapy, structural interventions require the creation of completely new functionings, a more comprehensive narrative of the events of the past and the reactivation of love for life and for one's parents.

A constant training to crystallize new decisions and to re-experiment new behaviors in the here and now.

It requires a very accurate and slow work that demands discipline, attention, determination, and great patience.

Persons let go of their defenses when they understand deeply that they were at the beginning princes and princesses and they can return to being them.

They can therefore try to find more adequate behaviors and in the meantime give themselves the permission to cry or be angry or afraid in the arms of someone.

These are already different behaviors and the revelation of modes of expression that had been inhibited until then.

From my vantage point I can say that in our progressively cold society that lacks socialization but is rich in sexual hints and deprived of love, oriented to success for gaining power and superfluous riches, deviated toward the greedy collection of refined and elitist pleasures, persons feel less and less oriented to express their belonging drive and to build relations based on love.

This is the reason why I care so much about this: we all lack it.

This is why in my treatments patients are often accompanied to relive and accept their fragility, a condition where human beings truly risk to break down when it is not accepted, comforted, shared, and overcome: the fragility of solitude, apathy and indifference.

It is not easy to kill a man – as historian Rutger Bregman (2019) has shown in his eye-opening last book – not to say a woman or a child, it is not easy to exploit them, enslave them, abuse them.

One needs first to somehow "go crazy" and become insensitive, be totally anesthetized from the sense of belonging and not consider the other a human being.

This psychic process is what "civilizations" have had to go through more or less recently to enslave or destroy large ethnic groups.

Not to feel the imperative, so dear to many religious and military and managerial groups, is one of the most serious damages dangerous for human beings.

And it is more and more often that in treatment we have to deal with the injunction DO NOT FEEL.

I remember a woman many years ago. From the very first sessions she had started to cry, she is my tears record woman, at least until now. After a few months she joined a group and cried all sessions through, when she came to residential groups she started crying at the very first exercises and cried for a couple of days. This lasted for about a year. She listened to what the others were working on and was moved by it.

And she wasn't whining; she cried soaked in tears.

In the meantime she went on with her usual life as a professional, a wife, and a mother.

I was young then and I remember I was very worried but my supervisor at the time, Alberto Torre, reassured me by writing "When persons are able to express their emotions they are not in danger, restraining is dangerous". I still keep that note among my most cherished quotations.

She was a person that had been "strong" for 45 years. She had grown in a family where she had never been a child, her mother had always needed her and she had never had a childhood and a youth, she had never been careless and had married a cold man, a good person but silent and distant, like her father (what a coincidence!) and now her father was dying. A father she had had no love relations with, a faraway man on whom she had not been able to pour her love.

She had quite a lot of tears to let out now that she was starting to understand what she had missed.

But she did not cry for the impending death of her very old father, she cried for not having been able to express her love for her father when she was a child and girl. During treatment she had understood and perceived, even only by getting in touch with the permission to feel, that it was time for her to let her Child part abandon the defensive pattern held for all her life in order to let herself feel her love for her father.

All the members of that group will always remember what she did to prepare her farewell to her dying father.

First she expressed all her anger against him because he had never seen or protected her as a child, then she wrote him a letter where she finally expressed her love and with the whole group around her she told her final goodbye to him.

After that preventative goodbye when she went to visit her father she hugged him as she had never been allowed to do while he, surprised, trying to brush her away, was visibly very happy.

When he finally died she barely cried. She was ready to let him go since she had finally been able to love him. Her treatment was made of many tears but also a lot of humanity.

One can let go in peace when love has been expressed fully.

When the real pain for what one has missed comes, persons stop pitying themselves, if they used to do it, they stop being angry at the world, stop pretending to be STRONG, PERFECT, PLEASING, stop living in a HURRY, stop TRYING HARD to do what they don't love, and finally cry with plenty of tears for what has not been, they cry the tears they have not shed in the past for their parents' inabilities that are now evident and understandable. It's their Child part crying.

And while they cry for their unexpressed love, they often cry also for their parents' unhappiness and for that relation that had not been loving for them too.

They cry because they could not love their parents how they are learning to do now with the compassion and sympathy that they are receiving from the group for their limits, faults and mistakes.

Yes, mistakes, how many mistakes can be understood while reading one's past anew!

And, if they understand their own mistakes and those of other group members, why shouldn't they understand their parents' too?

And in the end, can we call "mistakes" life courses that were so inevitable?

Behind these limits there are the limits of humankind and the defaults of the environments where we lived.

The limits of generations that only recently and in clearly defined privileged areas of the planet can have the goal of the pursuit of happiness and peace beyond a mere, often belligerent, survival.

As I was saying at the beginning, there are limits to our mind that is so developed but also so delicate in front of the responsibility that we took up to colonize the earth and be masters of our destiny, push away death and suffering and become "co-creators of the universe".

It's incredible how, when I ask a patient to impersonate a parent, they recover from their memory the same words and emotions that that parent offered to their child, like in Duilio's case, patients have not forgotten that tragedy ongoing in themselves, when they did not act it all their life long.

The sentence that can emerge, for example "go away and leave me alone" or "take care of me", "go against you father", "be nice to me", "win for me", and so on, when patients hear them re-emerging colored with their parent's emotions, become unacceptable and unbearable. Finally.

From the pain felt for having lived these tragedies as innocent children begins the true change.

Suffering indicates what must not happen "ever again".

This is why it is difficult to reject one's parents; if the disaster derived from not having been welcomed for what I am, and if this rejection must never be repeated in my life, how can I reject my parents and not be understanding with them?

So, when it is possible, we love again or at least commiserate.

The perception of pain, also of physical pain, is always a driver to change the state that caused it, pain is a spur to change. This is why we should feel it.

What person of sound mind would say it would be better not to feel any pain when one gets burned?

But there's more I would like to say about pain and the fear it often elicits. Pain is part of our life and if we always try to keep it at bay by trying to live healthily and happily, we cannot always avoid it.

In the end, when patients understand that in other circumstances their life could have been different, they feel real sadness for the lost chances, for the unexchanged love and for the time gone.

This pain is inevitable if not by accepting it as a part of our imperfect, fragile, sickly nature that no treatment will ever be able to change.

Treatment can also help to learn and accept and live all inevitable sorrows.

There is a video that can be found on the internet where the friends of a South African woman (https://www.youtube.com/watch?v=rGhrgesWqXE) who lost her hair after chemotherapy decide to shave their heads in sympathy. We see their reactions at the hairdresser's and it almost looks like a party; they laugh and joke and celebrate and a few are afraid: there is fear, surprise, and wonder in seeing themselves bald. Then they get ready to meet their friend and they shoot another video and take pictures there.

When the friend sees them all together, all bald like her, she is dumbstruck, she is obviously moved, they all kiss and hug in a climate of huge joy, friendship and love. They take pictures and raise glasses in a toast.

Their gazes are bright and happy. Happy in a moment of great sorrow.

A joy that pain can feel, sustain and welcome within itself.

I was uncertain whether to talk here about my own life. It seems that self-disclosures are not supposed to be present in an essay but then I thought that some of my experiences have taught me so much that it would be a pity to keep them to myself.

And so many years have passed that I think I can talk about them.

My first wife died of leukemia, a serious form due almost certainly to a previous chemotherapy undergone to fight a tumor.

But when I think of happiness I cannot but think of her gaze and her joy when, during her first stay in the special sterile ward, I went to see her clad from head to foot in protective clothing and she waved her cell phone at me and told me with great joy that she had received 70 texts.

I swear I never saw her happier in my life and we had been a happy couple for 35 years.

We hugged almost dancing and we knew very well that her leukemia could be deadly.

Then she read all the texts to me, one by one, and we marveled at some words and some persons from whom we didn't expect such warmth. We sat on her bed and smiled with tears in our eyes.

Other unexpected things happened in contact with that fear and that sorrow. I remember that we had become unable to watch TV: too many fights in talk shows, too much violence and blood in movies and serials, too much useless chatter.

With the TV off we were unconsciously cleansing ourselves.

We were purifying our souls and our bodies.

Our emotions were showing through our skin and all the rest seemed like *knickknack*.

The lives of other people changed too because they included a visit to that hospital ward in their daily lives: for five months they would come to spend some time with her. We had a carnet of visitors like the ball cards of the debutantes in old novels where they wrote the names of the young men they were to dance with, a list of the names and hours of our visitors.

Obviously my wife had her favorites, apart from me, as I was free to come at any time, the others had a ranking and we put some persons always at the same time in order to neutralize them so we included those with pitiful and sad looks, those who thought we were desperate and those who couldn't find words to say and lacked joy.

But we were deeply grateful to all when they entered the sterile room all clad in those funny caps and masks.

There has never been as much intimacy as in that period of our lives.

Months at the hospital, months of visits, and every day there were two hours of smiles, gazes, little presents, meetings. The eyes of persons were incredible, magnified by the masks that covered the rest of their faces, they contained everything, their hearts were exposed there.

The meetings were always joyful, with moments of chatting, telling stories of one's life and sharing, even when we were just playing cards silently, that silence was full of friendship.

No one ever talked of useless things. There wasn't much time, we couldn't waste a minute, and no one wanted to be elsewhere, which certainly is a measure of happiness and wellbeing.

She obviously lived for those hours while I left to give the others the full attention of the queen.

I was more or less a chamberlain, a handyman, an attendant, I went to collect persons and drove them back home, I talked to doctors and nurses and looked over all the movements and I never felt as important in my life.

Now I know that in those months when pain and fear were there, we felt also frequent moments of happiness.

What was going on? Do you have an answer?

We know how to find joy, we look for it in love, in self-assertion, in knowledge, in creativity, in growing a rose garden, we buy a dog because it makes us happy when it runs to us and licks our hands waving its tail. All beautiful things.

We know (many not clearly) how to be happy and how to make others happy in many ways but I assure you that in that room there were persons we did not let in because they didn't know how to suffer, what to do with pain, they weren't able to bring a drop of joy or sympathy or comfort.

Only embarrassment that is precisely the difficulty in showing one's emotions.

I remember once at a friend's funeral someone read a farewell speech that moved everybody, we were crying while that person was reading and we kept crying when we walked out of the church and hugged each other and we were happy, truly happy!

What makes us joyful together in certain moments? Is it actual happiness? Even during a funeral?

In a ward in a great hospital I read this notice: "*Joy draws people close, pain unites them!*"

Is this then that makes us happy? To feel united?

The managers of that hospital told me they had the habit of making nurses take turns and change wards to provide them with greater opportunities of professional growth and easier times, but they said it was very difficult to transfer the nurses of the cancer wards even if it meant a better position. They were all so proud of working there where the most seriously ill patients or children were staying because they said that life there is different.

Those who work in those wards feel important because they have a crucial and unique role in the life of others.

I don't think it's for generosity; I think that in some workplaces there is an enhancement of something that all humans have inside them: sympathy, self-realization, the wish "to count" for others or together with others.

And when this happens, we feel the deepest joy, as if suffering were the human condition that really unites us in our guts.

I also gave myself that answer: "Joy draws people close, pain unites them" much more than success, victory or conquest.

But probably it is also a different joy, less explosive, less energetic, less blinding, but certainly more intense, more permanent, deeper, and therefore more uniting.

Is it not in these moments that we need others most?

Those doctors and nurses live in a thick and intense dramatic atmosphere, but on that stage every day they enact a human drama of extraordinary intensity and meaning.

They feel they are very important, they realize their worth and put it in what they do and in general they receive a thankful recognition from patients and their relatives.

Most of all, they feel they have a very high goal, that their lives have a sacred task, to support persons in difficulty: they feel they are *essential*. They don't do their work as if it were just job for surviving. To survive the human condition needs the closeness and sharing generated by the deepest true joy.

And this is at times also the joy felt in therapeutic groups.

This applies also to us, how many of us psychotherapists would leave our places of distress and neurosis?

It seems to me that we don't leave them and we are attached to them all our lives long if we are able to see them as places of closeness, rebirth, change, and joy.

Both when we reach a success and when we share pain.

Like in that beautiful movie called "Departures" (https://en.wikipedia.org/wiki/Departures_(2008_film)).

It is the story of a musician that happens to become a mortician in Japan.

His work consists in preparing corpses, the "departed", for their funeral.

The movie describes his work course. At the beginning he is reluctant because he landed on the job by chance, he feels like a failure, rejected by society, and people treat him as such, even his wife is ashamed of that job and leaves him because that is the lowliest of jobs for all.

But slowly, as he learns from his master the precise, respectful, sweet actions necessary for doing the job well, this unpracticed and clumsy young man finds a way to create a state of grace in the room where the dead person's relatives collect for the ceremony of dressing the corpse.

Even when the departures are crushing and full of resentment, slowly, with the elegance, respect, care, and sacrality of his actions he can bring back all the persons present to a state that I felt corresponded to the state of nature.

Because something ancestrally unites humans in distress, especially in the face of something as deep and mysterious as death.

At that moment smiles form and an old feeling of sympathy is throbbing: co-belonging and closeness, in pain as in fear, alleviate suffering.

When a hand holds ours, we cannot but smile if we see a friendly human face near us.

A person, during a residential therapy group, was lying on the floor, tortured by grief for the recent loss of her partner and was sobbing quietly.

I moved near her in silence without touching her.

She felt I was near and after a while opened her sorrowful eyes. But it was a moment and when our eyes met she smiled, a smile I will always carry in my heart.

Later, when she was telling this event, she said it had been one of the most beautiful moments in her life and the same was for me.

Illness, suffering and death itself must not choke our joy of living; on the contrary. We must not let it happen.

Because the joy of living, of being in the world, cannot but include also suffering.

On the contrary, to be able to suffer, to be able to live facing pain, complements and exalts the joy of living.

After my wife's death I felt a great responsibility to be healthy and live even better the time that she no longer had to be happy. I learned never to waste it.

We should learn to live the pain in life in a different way, we would need a school! A school that teaches first of all the joy of living, always!

One can be happy and sad in the same day, not at the same time, but also in the most difficult conditions for a human being.

We need a school to teach us to feel pain to the full, because if we don't feel pain we won't feel joy and the wish and "duty" to be happy.

A school that teaches us that fragility does not mean weakness.

A school that teaches us that sooner or later some of the pain that is necessary to be full human beings will come our way.

The true challenge is to keep the joy of living even if we "must" suffer.

For five months inside and outside a leukemia ward my wife and I lived some of the most intense and beautiful moments of our life; they were also the most painful but, without being aware of it, she gave to all of us, relatives and friends and colleagues, thousands of reasons to give the best of ourselves in this life.

After her death, as she had requested, I organized a sort of happy hour where we talked about her, both crying and having fun.

I shied away from it when she suggested it, I still hoped she might recover and be healed, but when the moment came, I did what she asked me.

I put all the pictures of her I had in a big basket, whoever came in looked at them all, many crying but then smiling.

They then wrote notes containing some reflections or comments and put them in another basket. I still keep them jealously. All those notes thanked her for those few months of intense closeness.

They thanked her!

Paraphrasing the beautiful title of a book by Michela Marzano, *What Should We Do with Our Wounds?* (2012), I want to state that being close to a suffering person without avoiding our own painful emotions and those of others helps us live our life with the intensity it deserves, a life where every breath is a gift, every day a chance one should not waste.

Maybe it is not only a question of "What should we do with our wounds?" but what do we do while we are wounded.

When we are wounded we can exalt a part of ourselves, the attachment drive.

We are fragile but if we are together we will never feel weak.

On the contrary, since we know we are fragile, we try to find help in a moment of need and we stand together with others not to feel weak, not to feel anxious, not to be depressed, to be able to face all difficulties. And when we succeed we are happy.

We always look for each other in a storm, we hold hands and look up in order to wear on our breasts the word "dignity".

We have the same fate in common.

A therapy group is for me that school where we learn to face pain, the real and inevitable one.

Where pain feeds joy because it exalts it when it finally comes but also where the joy of living and being in the world allows us also to face pain.

Where we can feel OK also for the old suffering we have been able to turn into a road to rebirth.

Where we are also happy because we are together and give each other a hand to heal forever the wounds of old abandonment, indifference, violence, apathy, lack of love, loneliness, because we help each other to grow again like we were at the beginning, princes and princesses.

## Bibliography

Bregman R. (2019) *De meeste mensen deugen: een nieuwe geschiedenis van de mens* (Humankind: A Hopeful History). Amsterdam, De Correspondent BV.

Groddeck G. (1919) *Der Seelensucher. Ein psychoanalytischer Roman* (*The Seeker of Souls*). Lipsia/Vienna/Zurigo, Internationaler Psychoanalytischer Verlag.

Karpman S. (1968) Fairy tales and script drama analysis. In *Transactional Anayisis Bulletin*, 7(26): 39–43.

Cosso A. (2013) *Raccontarsela. Copioni di vita e storie organizzativ* (*Telling Yourself the Same Story Over and Over Again. Life Scripts and Organizational Narratives*). Milano, Lupetti.

Marzano M. (2012) *Cosa fare delle nostre ferite?* (*What to Do With Our Wounds?*). Trento, Erickson.

# Chapter 13

# Time Regained

I love my father – I write it in the present tense – because I started loving him again from the day of my uncle's great revelation, and I don't want to stop anymore.

It was a shock and I didn't need any psychotherapy then to realize the meanness and narrowness of my child gaze.

I was really ashamed because I had not understood that my father had effected a huge change in his life and had done it all by himself: grown up in violence he had found in religion a way not to repeat it.

He grew up with a rough and uncaring father, prone to abandonment and angry, and had done his best to prepare me to a future better than his.

He had been very demanding with me but because he cared for me, he wanted me to have a degree because he could not get one and had suffered in a menial job that brought him numberless humiliations.

He had even found a secure job at a bank for me because at the time in his opinion it was the best I could hope for.

While I thought only of playing football and hid comics inside my schoolbooks.

That day something happened inside me that I see always happening in those who reconcile themselves with their parents.

We remember the rest.

When we are angry at our parents we children remember only their bad deeds, we have such a selective perception that they become ogres and witches and we always look at all they do with a focused critical gaze ready to select the worst.

Without reconstructing the story of our lives, without a historical view of what came before us everything remains indistinct and confused, our past like our present with the influences that affected us.

In the end we no longer know who we are and what distinguishes us from our parents.

Children's opinions are affected by the conclusions they draw from what they see, and if they see their father harassing their mother, he is clearly the bad

DOI: 10.4324/9781003303831-13

guy and she is the good one. What do they know of what it was like between them in reality?

Or, on the contrary, she is certainly evil and doesn't take care of him enough.

But if we cannot expect a systemic view from a child, it is when we grow up that we must widen our gaze and include that background from which we extracted what we needed to understand life or to take a side.

For me, as for many others, to bring the background to the forefront has been a revelation.

My father was a father, harsh and fair, inflexible and grieving, bad and good, at times he gave me a little money if I behaved well.

He always came to see me when I played important matches, and when he was free from work he took me to practice and if I got bad grades or came home late from the playing field (both occurring quite frequently) he would send me to bed without dinner.

But since that meeting with my uncle, I started remembering also the rest.

I remembered that on the side of the playing field the coach was sitting on a bench with the masseur and the other kids. On the other side stood my father, outside the fence giving me advice and yelling: "Forestall, Giorgio, move, anticipate!".

And still today I never miss a train or plane, I am never late, I arrive early.

I remembered an episode that I had completely forgotten, one of the few moments when he showed understanding of my problems at school. He had come to my finals and saw me very anxious and confused trying to answer math questions.

That night at home he told me that he didn't care if I did not pass, he saw how difficult it had been for me, but he knew I had tried my best and it was evident that the teacher was trying to make me fall in a trap while I tried to answer as best as I could.

I remembered that a few years later he had told me that the principal of the school had advised him not to make me go on studying because he thought I was not fit for university but my father, despite his respect for authorities, had not believed him.

I had totally forgotten this sign of immense and tenacious trust in me that did not correspond with my idea of him when I was young.

I never thought he had a high opinion of me; he was the kind of man that talks well of you only to strangers (and I didn't hear that), while to me he always said I was not proficient and almost good for nothing (and this I did hear).

I remembered that my father used to cry when he watched moving scenes on TV and when the Pope sent his blessing "urbi et orbi".

I remember that when I was a boy he used to take me to football games and tried not to make me pay for the ticket by hiding me first behind him and then before him with a protective gesture. I can still feel his hands on my shoulders guiding me through the crowd and skirting the guy checking the tickets.

I remembered that together we siphoned the wine from the demijohn to the bottles (I still do it and will do it for the rest of my life). We sucked the tube and inserted it swiftly in the bottles but at the end of the process I was slightly tipsy, and he too, and we laughed.

But with this he was teaching me how to calculate times and certain practical crafts that could then be transferred to the mind.

He liked to teach me how to do things well.

I remembered that he paid board and lodging for me to attend university in a different city from ours and when I threatened to study and work in order to choose the subject I wanted (I was as stubborn as he was) he indignantly said "Don't even think of doing that! Think of studying and I take care of letting you get your degree!"

He didn't realty trust me that much and thought I wouldn't make it, but he did all he could to make me study, while I did all I wanted away from home and from him. And I considered him a tyrant.

I think this was the reason why at the university I started studying seriously and I graduated with honors.

I remembered that he had a high sense of justice, helped the poor, worked as a volunteer, was active in his church and managed the parish cinema.

And I adore cinema and organize a film forum for the students of our school for therapists.

And I never heard him quarreling with my mother.

He tried all means to convince me of his religious and political ideas and never succeeded but in more recent years he even started listening to my arguments.

In the end, even if with his threatening gaze on my shoulders, I did what I wanted and autonomy has never been a problem for me.

I remembered that once, while I should have been studying at college, he saw me in the news at a political gathering in Rome, 600 kilometers away from where I said I was.

He made me go home and asked me to explain what I was doing there, and I told him it was the founding of a group of Christians for Socialism.

The word *Christian* was enough to make him overlook the word *Socialism* and he only said: "The next time tell us before you go if you don't want to scare the light out of your mother!"

The surprising thing is that all these paternal attitudes (but the same happens also with mothers) when unseen remain on the background also in our adult life, we simply don't know we have them but when we become aware of them then we notice them all the time.

When we truly make peace then we can see and appreciate them.

So, when I learned to love my father, I discovered in myself another part of my Parent Ego State.

An assertive, constant, strong, protective parent that exposes himself and fights.

And is demanding, very demanding.

A student recently told me that I am a teacher of "rules" and "smiles". I must have joined my father and mother in this.

A parent that almost always says what he thinks but also lets his children do, remaining protectively at a distance, like him.

With my students, with my patients, and even with my children, among a great many uncertainties and doubts, suddenly my parental automatisms found their way: my outrage for badly done jobs, my being demanding and not giving up in front of difficulties, my anger against injustice and against tax dodgers, my attention for things and even a new respect toward authorities; they were all his qualities.

To reject his flaws, that I saw much larger than they were, was always easy but to take possession of his qualities was much more difficult and all started when I became aware of the extraordinary evolutionary passage that he had been able to accomplish without anyone's help.

Those parental competences in me were dampened and unseen.

From that famous day on every time I went to visit my parents I saw him with different eyes, I noticed his attitudes with total benevolence and I started hugging and kissing him and he was always surprised that I did.

I filled the distance that he had created from his Natural Child part that he had had to leave in his native village, cancelled first by fear and later by a repetitive and often humiliating job.

His efforts at becoming a man, becoming "a respectable citizen" had been huge, with a world war to fight, no family, no money, brought up by an old countryside priest.

How can one not love a father like him?

But so are many persons, and I too.

My story is not as tragic as the stories I hear from my patients, but the mechanisms that govern the perception of our story and its narrative are the same, just like the sense of peace and fulfillment that warms our hearts when interrupted filial love is reactivated.

For many patients the end of therapy coincides with this stage.

Love for the Other is reactivated at a different level, we no longer love because nature and blood make us do it, nor because during childhood we had to be close to those who generated us.

That love changes because we recovered the urge to love life, because we reconciled with our "origin".

We no longer love for surviving or simply for fulfilling the belonging drive, no longer just for attachment, to have a family, to have a partner in life.

No, we love now because we know how to love and we revitalized at last the natural urge that is the origin of the continuation of our species.

That ancestral drive that is held back when our first experiences have been frustrating is now free and allows us to look at the world with new eyes, not those of the child we have been, innocent and pure, before the great frost set in, but those of today that have finally shed the fear of not being welcome and the suspicion of not being OK.

Our eyes today can no longer be innocent and pure but can still be trusting and available.

The difference between them and the loving gaze of a newborn is that we now know more about the world, we know that all persons love for what they have received and for what they have been taught, we know Evil exists and the deterioration of the mind, we know that we have to be careful and protect ourselves, but, most of all, we know that we must not let ourselves be corrupted and spoil the precious good that is in ourselves, original and universal, that makes us happy more than anything else.

The disposition to Good – the original blessing (Fox, 1983), the passion principle (Mancuso, 2013), the substantial goodness of human beings (Bregman, 2019) – is the aspiration of every human being to live in harmony with the world. It is also for this reason that the belonging drive is an integral part of the survival drive because without harmony, love, con-sonance, our life would end and with it our species.

We love our parents not because of a commandment, not because we must, not because we pity older people, we love them for the equanimity deriving from the discovery of what human nature is in all persons, even those that we consider psychopaths or perverts or jerks or losers, including witches and ogres.

I find it difficult to think that one can be a good therapist without being at peace with one's internal fathers and mothers.

So that there is no longer an actively looming parent threatening our minds with their miseries.

Only a pale memory of that story will remain but it will no longer affect us

As in Giulia's tale that terrorized her as a child only because she was held in the arms of a scared mother.

As in Duilio's tale where a mother seemed to kick out her helpless and awkward son while she "only" hated herself and her life and wanted to save him by sending him away from her.

At last we are free to look at the difficulties near the merits, free to feel that we are children of that original good of each species, free from the original sin of a monstrous family that actually wasn't that monstrous and therefore we aren't monstrous either.

That family wasn't that hateful if we are here alive and talk about it in treatment, intelligent, reflective, moved, and sound enough in mind and body to try to be different from them and even happy.

And our nature cannot be less than Good.

This is the new narrative that science has been showing us in the past few years. (Fox, 1983, Eibl-Eibessfeldt, 1989, Sen, 1999, Ehrlich, 2000, Dunbar, 2014, 2020, De Waal, 2009, 2013, Tomasello, 2009, Brooks, 2011, Sennet, 2012, Diamond, 2012, Mancuso, 2013, Bloom, 2013, Pievani, 2014, Bregman, 2019, and many others).

Before closing I would like to add a last crucial reflection that I also consider necessary: we have been taught that human beings need recognitions, adequate feedback, to build their identity and we grow and individuate in this way.

Our identity is a social gift because the others send back to us what we are all life long, but until when?

Should we continue for all our life to depend from the recognition of our deeds; should we continue for all our life to ask if what we do is well done, waiting for a visible response from others?

Do we always have to wait and see if the others and society reward our behaviors?

Or is it possible for a layperson, without following any religious precept, to tell themselves "well done".

Is there a for nature and an against nature that can orient our course every day, our work all life long?

Maybe at a certain age we can stop looking for recognitions and learn a new natural sensitivity that still checks its operations with others but takes on responsibility for its own choices?

What is good for a human being?

In therapy groups we always ask What does us good and what harms us?

What's good for this moment in my life and what is good for you?

We realize always that each patient has their own drive to recover to complete their "humanity" that is in all that common denominator that satisfies and gives joy, that feeds and rewards and that needs no other recognition or approval but only understanding and acceptance.

We don't need gifts or rewards after making love.

We don't need good marks after learning something useful and interesting.

The same applies to a good swim in the sea, to writing a poem or reading a good book.

After these joys, that are essential and depend on drives, we need no further "pleasure" or reward.

That virtue rewards itself has been said by many, lay and religious persons. Socrates was probably the first one along with stoics: "virtue is in itself the harbinger of happiness in the serene and unassailable self-awareness of the righteous".

Then Epicurean philosophers, then Pietro Pomponazzi, who risked burning at the stake in the late 1500s for stating that "to behave virtuously one does not need to believe in the immortality of souls and rewards in heaven because virtue is a reward in itself".

Is there a virtue that we can listen to only in the depth of our guts?

I think that in psychotherapeutic group work there is often a spiritual value added that does not seem ideological to me. We are together to help each other rediscover our "good" nature, to maintain and reconquer the joy of living both in happiness and in sorrow.

We are together to remove the damper that prevented sorrow from indicating to us what was wrong for our nature.

We are together to acknowledge that there are no mistakes or faults but only the inevitable consequences of abuse, harassment, indifference, invasion, that in turn came from a past damage, repeated millions of times for millions of years before it reached us.

We are together not to confess mistakes or guilt but to accept our limits with dignity and look openly at them to try to evolve a little more.

We are together to learn to be together and give value to belonging.

We are together to be healthy and happy.

As I said, we need to preserve our nature to defend what is good for us, for our children, for our communities, for our species.

Let's stop slandering humans.

We only need to evolve naturally as we discover that the adaptations, opinions and behaviors of the past no longer work.

And there are always new Permissions to try to realize as much as possible in a community that for which we have been brought to the world.

Because each one of us has been brought to the world, we are the gift our species gives to itself, each newborn is the hope for a better world but we have to be able to go beyond what has been done of us by those who came before us.

Life is not a gift made to us. Life is not given to us, as is commonly said.

We are brought to the world.

We are the gift, as Raimon Panikkar (2005) taught us, given to life, the one that was before us and will continue after us for a long time.

Let us then unwrap this gift, let's take the wrappings off, let's throw away paper and ribbons and take out what is beautiful inside: our love for life and original humanity.

Bloom – is Result – to meet a Flower And casually glance
Would scarcely cause [one] to suspect the minor Circumstance
Assisting in the Bright Affair So intricately done
Then offered as a Butterfly To the Meridian –
To pack the Bud – oppose the Worm – Obtain its right of Dew –
Adjust the Heat – elude the Wind – Escape the prowling Bee
Great Nature not to disappoint Awaiting Her that Day –
To be a Flower, is profound Responsibility –

Emily Dickinson

From *Bolts of Melody: New Poems of Emily Dickinson*. Edited by Mabel Loomis Todd and Millicent Todd Bingham. New York: Harper & Brothers Publishers.

## Bibliography

Bloom P. (2013) *Just Babies: The Origins of Good and Evil*. New York, The Crown Publishing Group.

Bregman R. (2019) *De meeste mensen deugen: een nieuwe geschiedenis van de mens* (*Humankind: A Hopeful History*). Amsterdam, De Correspondent BV.

Brooks D. (2011) *The Social Animal: The Hidden Sources of Love, Character, and Achievement*. New York, Random House.

De Waal F. (2009) *The Age of Empathy: Nature's Lessons for a Kinder Society*. New York, Harmony Books.

De Waal F. (2013) *The Bonobo. And the Atheist: In Search Ok Humanism Among the Primates*. New York, W. W. Norton & Company.

Diamond J. (2012) *The World until Yesterday: What Can We Learn from Traditional Societies?* London, Penguin Books.

Dickinson E. (1945) *Bolts of Melody: New Poems of Emily Dickinson*. Edited by Mabel Loomis Todd and Millicent Todd Bingham. New York, Harper & Brothers Publishers.

Dunbar R. (2011) *How Many Friends Does One Person Need?* London, Faber & Faber.

Dunbar R. (2014) *Human Evolution*. London, Penguin Books.

Dunbar R. (2020) *Evolution. What Everyone Needs to Know*. New York, Oxford University Press.

Ehrlich P. (2000) *Human Natures: Genes, Cultures, and the Human Prospect*. Washington, D.C., Island Press for Shearwater Books.

Eibl-Eibessfeldt I. (1989) *Human Ethology*. New York, Routledge.

Fox M. (1983) *The Original Blessing*. Rochester, Vermont, Bear & Co.

Mancuso V. (2013) *Il principio passione. (The Passion Principle)*. Milano, Garzanti.

Panikkar R. (2005) *La dimora della saggezza (The Abode of Wisdom)*. Milano, Mondadori.

Pievani T. (2014) *Evoluti e abbandonati. (Evolved and Abandoned)*. Torino, Einaudi.

Sen, Amartya. (2000) *Development as Freedom*. New York, Anchor.

Sennet R. (2012) *Together: The Rituals, Pleasures and Politics of Cooperation*. London, Yale University Press.

Tomasello M. (2009) *Why We Cooperate*, Cambridge, MA, MIT Press.

# Full Bibliography

Alberini C., Travaglia A. (2017) Infantile amnesia: A critical period of learning to learn and remember. In *The Journal of Neuroscience*, Jun 14; 37(24): 5783–5795.

Allemandri D., Baldacci M., Ciurli M. P., Poidomani S., Procacci M. A., Salnitro P., (2012) *Bisogni spezzati, bisogni ritrovati. Nuovi orizzonti di analisi transazionale elaborati nella bottega di Carlo Moiso* (*Broken Needs. Rediscovered Needs. New Horizons of Transactional Analysis Developed in the Workshop of Carlo Moiso*). Roma, Alpes Italia Ed.

Ammaniti M. (2014) *Noi. Perché due sono meglio di uno* (*We. Why two is better than one*). Bologna, Il Mulino.

Ammaniti M., Gallese V. (2014) *The Birth of Intersubjectivity. Psychodynamic, Neurobiology, and Self*. New York, W. W. Norton & Co.

Arendt H. (1963) *Eichmann in Jerusalem: A Report on the Banality of Evil*. Viking Press.

Balint M. (1985) *Primary Love and Psychoanalytic Technique*. New York, Routledge.

Balint M. (1992) *The Basic Fault: Therapeutic Aspects of Regression*. Evanston, Illinois U.S. Northwestern University Press.

Baumann Z. (2005) *Liquid life*. Cambridge, Polity Press.

Baumann Z. (2013) *Le sorgenti del male*. (*The Origins of Evil*). Trento, Erickson.

Baumeister R. F., Leary M. R. (1995) The need to belong: Desire for interpersonal attachments as a fundamental human motivation. In *Psychological Bulletin*, 117: 497–529.

Berne E. (1947) *The Mind in Action. A Layman's Guide to Psychiatry and Psychoanalisys*. New York, Simon and Schuster.

Berne E. (1961) *TA in Psychotherapy*. New York, Grove Press.

Berne E. (1964) *Games People Play*. New York, Grove Press.

Berne E. (1966) *Principles of Group Treatment*. New York, Oxford University Press.

Berne E. (1970) *Sex in Human Loving*. London, Penguin.

Berns G. (2005) *Satisfaction: The Science of Finding True Fulfillment*. New York, Henry Holt & Co. Inc.

Bloom P. (2013) *Just Babies: The Origins of Good and Evil*. New York, The Crown Publishing Group.

Bollas C. (1982) On the relation to the self as an object. In *The International Journal of Psychoanalysis*, 63(3): 347–359.

Boncinelli E. (2000) *Le forme della vita. L'evoluzione e l'origine dell'uomo* (*Life Forms. Evolution and the Origin of Man*). Torino, Einaudi.

Borgna E. (2001) *L'arcipelago delle emozioni* (*The Archipelago of Emotions*). Milano, Feltrinelli.

Borgna E. (2013) *La dignità ferita* (*The Wounded Dignity*). Milano, Feltrinelli.

Borgogno F. (2009) *La partecipazione affettiva dell'analista. Il contributo di Sandor Ferenczi al pensiero psicoanalitico contemporane* (*The Affective Participation of the Analyst. Sandor Ferenczi's Contribution to Contemporary Psychoanalytic Thought*). Torino, Codice Edizioni.

Bowlby J. (1979) *The Making and Breaking of Affectional Bonds*. London, Routledge.

Bowlby J. (1988) *A Secure Base: Parent-Child Attachment and Healthy Human Development*. New York, Basic Books.

Bregman R. (2019) *De meeste mensen deugen: een nieuwe geschiedenis van de mens* (*Humankind: A Hopeful History*). Amsterdam, De Correspondent BV.

Bromberg P. M. (1998) *Standing in the Spaces: Essays on Clinical Process Trauma and Dissociation*. New York, Taylor & Francis Group.

Brooks D. (2011) *The Social Animal: The Hidden Sources of Love, Character, and Achievement*. New York, Random House.

Cacciari M. (2015) *King Lear. Fathers, Sons, Heirs*. Caserta, Saletta dell'Uva.

Calzolaio V., Pievani T. (2016) *Libertà di migrare: Perché ci spostiamo sempre ed è bene così* (*Freedom to Migrate: Why We're Always Moving and It's Okay to Do So*). Torino, Einaudi.

Capitini A. (1956) *Colloquio corale* (*Choral Conversation*). Pisa, Pacini Mariotti.

Capra F. (1996) *The Web of Life*. New York, Doubleday.

Cavalli Sforza L., Menozzi P., Piazza A. (1994) *The History of Geography of Human Genes*. Princeton, NJ, Princeton University Press.

Cavalli Sforza L., Pievani T. (2011) *Homo sapiens. La grande storia della diversità umana* (*Homo sapiens. The grand story of human diversity*). Torino, Codice.

Clarkson P. (1992) Physis in transactional analysis. In *Transactional Analysis Journal*, 22: 202–209.

Coon C. (1946) The universality of natural groupings in human societies. In *The Journal of Educational Sociology*, 20(3): 163–168.

Cornell W. F. (1988) Life script theory: A critical review from a developmental perspective. In *Transactional Analysis Journal*, 18(4).

Cornell W. F. (2000) If Berne meet Winnicot: TA and relation analysis. In *TAJ*, 18: 4.

Cornell W. F. (2001) There ain't no cure without sex: The provision of a vital base. In *Transactional Analysis Journal*, 31: 233–239.

Cornell W. F. (2015) *Somatic Experience in Psichoanalysis and Psychotherapy: In the Expressive Language of the Living*. New York, Taylor & Francis Group.

Cornell W. F., De Graaf A., Newton T., Thunissen M. (2016) *Into TA. A Comprehensive Textbook on Transactional Analysis*. London, Karnac Book.

Cosso A. (2013) *Raccontarsela. Copioni di vita e storie organizzativ* (*Telling Yourself the Same Story Over and Over Again. Life Scripts and Organizational Narratives*). Milano, Lupetti.

Cosso A. (2014) Copione, narrazione, destino, identità, storytelling (Script, narrative, destiny, identity, storytelling). In *RIC Rivista Italiana di Counseling*, 1(1): 42–63.

Dalai Lama, Goleman D. (2003) *Destructive Emotions: A Scientific Dialogue with the Dalai Lama*. New York, Bantam Book.

Damasio A. (1994) *Descartes' Error: Emotion, Reason, and the Human Brain*. New York, Putnam.

Damasio A. (2003) *Looking for Spinoza: Joy, Sorrow, and the Feeling Brain*, San Diego, Harcourt.

Damasio A. (2010) *Feeling, Being, and Knowing: A Manifesto on Consciousness*. New York, Pantheon.

Damasio A. (2021) *Feeling and Knowing: Making Minds Conscious*. Boston: Little, Brown Book Group.

De Waal F. (1991) The chimpanzee's sense of social regularity and its relation to the human sense of justice. In *American Behavorial Scientist*, 34(3): 335–349.

De Waal F. (1996) *Good Natured: The Origins of Right and Wrong in Humans and Other Animals*. Cambridge US, Harvard University Press.

De Waal F. (2006) *Primates and Philosophers: How Morality Evolved*. Princeton, NJ, University Press.

De Waal F. (2009) *The Age of Empathy: Nature's Lessons for a Kinder Society*. New York, Harmony Books.

De Waal F. (2013) *The Bonobo. And the Atheist: In Search Ok Humanism Among the Primates*. New York, W. W. Norton & Company.

Deci E. L., Ryan R. M. (1985) *Intrinsic Motivation and Self-Determination in Human Behavior*. New York, Plenum Press.

Deci E. L., Ryan R. M. (2000) The "what" and "why" of goal pursuits: Human needs and the self-determination of behavior. In *Psychological Inquiry*, 11: 227–268.

Dehaene S. (2014) *Consciousness and the Brain: Deciphering How the Brain codes Our Thoughts*. New York, Viking Press.

Dehaene S., Duhamel J. R., Hauser M., Rizzolatti G. (2005) *From Monkey Brain to Human Brain*. Cambridge, MA, MIT Press.

Del Giudice E. (2007) Old and New Views on the Structure of Matter and the special case of Living Matter. In *Journal of Physics Conference Series*, 67: 012006.

Diamond J. (2012) *The World until Yesterday: What Can We Learn from Traditional Societies?* London, Penguin Books.

Dickinson E. (1945) *Bolts of Melody: New Poems of Emily*. Edited by Mabel Loomis Todd and Millicent Todd Bingham. New York: Harper & Brothers Publishers.

Dunbar R. (2011) *How Many Friends Does One Person Need?* London, Faber & Faber.

Dunbar R. (2014) *Human Evolution*. London, Penguin Books.

Dunbar R. (2020) *Evolution. What Everyone Needs to Know*. New York, Oxford University Press.

Ehrlich P. (2000) *Human Natures: Genes, Cultures, and the Human Prospect*. Washington, D.C., Island Press for Shearwater Books.

Eibl-Eibessfeldt I. (1989) *Human Ethology*. New York, Routledge.

Eibl-Eibessfeldt I. (1996) *Love and Hate*. New York, Routledge.

English F. (1976) Racketeering. In *Transactional Analysis Journal*, 6(1): 76–81.

English F. (1988) Whither script? In *Transactional Analysis Journal*, 18(4): 294–303.

English F. (1992) *Analyse Transactionnelle et Emotions*. (Transactional analysis and emotions). Paris, Desclée de Brouwer.

English F. (2008) What Motivates Resilience After Trauma? In *TAJ*, 38(4): 343–351.

English F. (2010) It Takes a Lifetime to Play Out a Script, In Erskine R. *Life Scripts: a Transactional Analysis of Unconscious Relational Patterns*. London, Karnac.

Erskine R. (2010) *Life Scripts: A Transactional Analysis of Unconscious Relational Patterns*. New York, Routledge.

Erskine R. G. (2013a) Relational group process. Development in a transactional analysis model of group psychotherapy. In *Transactional Analysis Journal*, 43(4): 262–275.

Erskine R. G. (2013b) Vulnerability, authenticity and inter-subjective contact: Philosophical principles of integrative psychotherapy. In *International Journal of Integrative Psychotherapy*, 2: 1–9.

Erskine R. G. (2019) *Transactional Analysis in Contemporary Psychotherapy*. New York: Routledge.

Erskine R. G. (2021) *A Healing Relationship: Commentary on Therapeutic Dialogues*. Bicester, Oxfordshire, Phoenix Publishing House.

Fantini M. (2009) *Analisi transazionale e neuroscienze. Un binomio da riscoprire* (*Transactional Analysis and Neuroscience. A Pair to Be Rediscovered*). Torino, Ananke.

Foster Wallace D. (2009) *This Is Water*. New York, Little, Brown and Company.

Fox M. (1983) *The Original Blessing*. Rochester, Vermont, Bear & Co.

Fraiberg Selma H. (1999) *Il sostegno allo sviluppo* (*Development support*). Milano, Raffaello Cortina.

Frankl V. (1969) *Man's Search Formeaning*. London, Hodder & Stoughton.

Fromm E. (1956) *The Art of Loving*, New York, Harper & Row.

Fromm E. (1992) *Humanismus als reale Utopie. Der Glaube an den Menschen* (*Humanism as a Real Utopia. The Belief in Man*). Weinheim GE, Beltz.

Galimberti U. (2002) *Psiche e techne. L'uomo nell'età della tecnica* (*Psiche and Techne. Man in the Age of Technology*). Milano, Feltrinelli.

Galimberti U. (2004) *Le cose dell'amore* (*Things of Love*). Milano, Feltrinelli.

Galimberti U. (2008) *La casa di psiche. Dalla psicoanalisi alla pratica filosofica* (*The House of Psyche. From Psychoanalysis to Philosophical Practice*). Milano, Feltrinelli.

Galimberti U. (2009a) *Paesaggi dell'anima* (*Landscapes of the Soul*). Milano, Mondadori.

Galimberti U. (2009b) *I miti del nostro tempo* (*The Myths of Our Time*). Milano, Feltrinelli.

Goulding R., Goulding M. (1976) Injunctions, decisions, and redecisions. In *Transactional Analysis Journal*, 6: 41–48.

Goulding R., Goulding M. (1979) *Changing Lives Through Redecision Therapy*. New York, Brunner/Mazel.

Gregoire J. (2007) *Les orientations rècentes de l'analyse transactionnelle* (*The new direction of transactional analysis*). Lyon, Les Editions d'Analys transactionelle.

Groddeck G. (1919) *Der Seelensucher. Ein psychoanalytischer Roman* (*The Seeker of Souls*). Lipsia/Vienna/Zurigo, Internationaler Psychoanalytischer Verlag.

Harari Y. N. (2014) *Sapiens: A Brief History of Humankind*. London, Harvill Secker.

Harari Y. N. (2016) *Homo Deus: A Brief History of Tomorrow*. London, Harvill Secker.

Hargaden H. E., Sills C. (2002) *Transactional Analysis: A Relational Perspective*. Hove, UK, Brunner-Routledge.

Harris T. H. (1969) *I'm OK – You're OK*. New York, Harper & Row.

Hay J. (2009) *Working It Out at Work; Understanding Attitudes and Building Relationships*. Watfoord, UK, Sherwood.

Hellinger B. (1998a) *Love's Hidden Symmetry. What Makes Love Work in Relationship*. Phoenix, AZ, Zeig, Tucker.

Hellinger B. (1998b) *Ordungen der Liebe* (*Orders of Love*). Heidelberg, Carl-Auer.

Hellinger B. (2001) *Love's Own Truths: Bonding and Balancing in Close Relationships*. Phoenix, Tucker & Theisen.

Hillman J. (1997) *The Soul's Code*. New York, Bantam.

Imbasciati A. (2005) *La sessualità e la teoria energetico pulsionale: Freud e le conclusioni sbagliate di un percorso geniale. (Sexuality and Drive Energy Theory: Freud and the Mistaken Conclusions of a Brilliant Path)*. Milano, Franco Angeli.

Janet P., Orbecchi M. (2014) *La psicoanalisi*. Torino, Bollati Boringhieri.

Kahler T. (2008) *The Process Therapy Model: The Six Personality Types with Adaptations*. Little Rock, AK, Taibi Kahler Associates.

Kahler T., Capers H. (1974) The miniscript. In *Transactional Analysis Journal*, 4(1): 26–42.

Karpman S. (1968) Fairy tales and script drama analysis. In *Transactional Anayisis Bulletin*, 7(26): 49–52.

Karpman S. (2009) Sex games people play: Intimacy blocks, games, and scripts. In *Transactional Analysis Journal*, 39(2): 103–116.

Karpman S (2010) Intimacy analysis today. The intimacy scale and the personality pinwheel. In *Transactional Analysis Journal*, 40(3–4): 224–242.

Klein M. (1983) *Discover Your Real Self*. London, Hutchinson & co.

Langer A. (1994) Quattro consigli per un futuro amico. (Four Tips for a Future Friend). In *Rocca*, 8-1995, Assisi, Cittadella di Assisi.

Langer A. (2011) *Il viaggiatore leggero. Scritti 1961 – 1995 (The Light Traveler)*. Palermo, Sellerio.

Le Doux J. (1996) *The Emotional Brain (The Mysterious Underpinnings of Emotional Life)*. New York, Simon & Schuster, Touchstone.

Levin P. (1988) *Cycles of Power*. Deerfield Beach, Fla., Health Communications.

Lichtenberg Joseph D. (1989) *Psychoanalysis and Motivation*. New York, Routledge.

Lowen A. (1958) *The Language of the Body*. New York, Collier Books.

Lowen A. (1975) *Bioenergetics*. New York, Coward, McCann & Geoghegan.

MacLean P. D. (1990) *The Triune Brain in Evolution (Role in Paleocerebral Functions)*. New York, Plenum Press.

Magrograssi G. (2014) *I gioche che giochiamo (The Games We Play)*. Milano, Baldini Castoldi.

Mancuso V. (2007) *L'anima e il suo destino (The Soul and Its Destiny)*. Milano, Raffaello Cortina.

Mancuso V. (2013) *Il principio passione. (The Passion Principle)*. Milano, Garzanti.

Marchino L. (1995) *La bioenergetica (Bioenergetics)*. Milano, Xenia.

Marchino L. (2015) *Risvegliare l'energia. (Awakening Energy)*. Milano, Mimesis.

Marchino L., Mizrahil M. (2011) *Il corpo non mente (The Body Does Not Lie)*. Milano, Pickwick.

Marinopulos S. (2005) *Dans l'intime des mères (In the innermost of mothers)*. Paris, Fayard.

Marzano M. (2012) *Cosa fare delle nostre ferite? (What to Do With Our Wounds?)*. Trento, Erickson.

Maslow A. (1954) *Motivation and Personality*. London, Harper & Row.

Mazzetti M. (2004) La supervisione. Scambi di saperi (Supervision. Exchanges of knowledge). *Quaderni di psicologia, Analisi transazionale e Scienze umane*, 42. Milano, La vita felice.

Mazzetti M. (2007) Supervision in transactional analysis: An operational model. In *Transactional Analysis Journal*, 37(2): 93–103.

Mazzetti M. (2013) Un sistema motivazionale per l'Analisi Transazionale. (A Motivational System for Transactional Analysis). In Berardo C. *Fanita English. Quaderno delle giornate di studio di Lavarone*. Torino, Zedde.

Mazzetti M. (2014) Petruska Clarkson Physis in AT, integrazioni e confronti (Petruska Clarkson Physis in AT integrations and comparisons) in *Quaderno delle Giornate di studio di Lavarone, ITACA*.

McNeel J. (1976) The Parent interview. *Transactional Analysis Journal*, 6, (1): 61–68.

Miller A. (1997) *The Drama of the Gifted Child: The Search for the True Self. Completely Revised and Updated With a New Afterword by the Author*. New York, Harper Collins.

Mitchell S. A. (1988) *Relational Concepts in Psychoanalysis: An Integration*. Cambridge, MA, Harvard University Press.

Mitchell S. A. (2001) *Can Love Last? The Fate of Romance Over Time*. New York, Norton.

Moiso C. (1998) Being and belonging. In *Script*, 28(9): 1–7.

Moiso C., Novellino M. (1982) *Stati dell'Io (Ego states)*. Roma, Astrolabio.

Niebuhr R. (1987) *The Essential Reinhold Niebuhr: Selected Essays and Addresses*. New haven, London, Yale University Press.

Novellino M. (2014) *Seminari berniani. La prassi dell'analisi transazionale. (Bernian Seminars. The Praxis of Transactional Analysis)*. Milano, F. Angeli.

Novellino M. (2016) *Psicoanalisi transazionale. Manuale di psicodinamica relazionale per psicoterapeuti e counselor. (Transactional Psychoanalysis. Handbook of Relational Psychodynamics for Psychotherapists and Counselors)*. Milano, F. Angeli.

Nowak M., Highfield R. (2011) *SuperCooperators: Altruism, Evolution, and Why We Need Each Other to Succeed*. New York, Free Press.

Orbecchi M. (2015) *Biologia dell'anima. Teoria dell'evoluzione e psicoterapia. (Biology of the Soul. Evolutionary Theory and Psychotherapy)*. Torino, Bollati Boringhieri.

Pagliarani L. (1985) *Il coraggio di Venere. Anti-manuale di psico-socio-analisi della vita presente. (The Courage of Venus. Anti-Manual of Psycho-Socio-Analysis of Present Life)*. Milano, Raffaello Cortina.

Panikkar R. (2005a) *La dimora della saggezza (The Abode of Wisdom)*. Milano, Mondadori.

Panikkar R. (2005b) *La nuova innocenza (The new innocence)*, Sotto il Monte (Bg), Servitium.

Panksepp J., Biven L. (2012) *The Archeology of Mind. New York. Neuroevolutionary Origins Of Human Emotions*. New York, W. W. Norton & Company.

Piccinino G. (2000) *La forza del destino (The Power of Destiny)*. Napoli, Dinosauro.

Piccinino G. (2006) *Il piacere di lavorare (The Pleasure of Working)*. Trento, Erickson.

Piccinino G. (2011a) Pulsioni innate e riconoscimenti, un contributo alla teoria del Copione. (Innate drives and recognition, a contribution to script theory). In *AT Rivista Italiana di Analisi Transazionale e metodologie terapeutiche*. xxx, n° 22/2010, Roma, Simpat.

Piccinino G. (2011b) We empowerment. In *Pagine Mida*. Milano, Fondazione Mida.

Piccinino G. (2012) La ferita dei non amaNti. (The wound of non-lovers). In *Neopsiche* N°12, Torino, Ananke.

Piccinino G. (2014) In principio c'è la natura: contributi dell'evoluzionismo al concetto di benessere. (In the beginning is nature: contributions of evolutionism to the concept of well-being.) In *RIC, Rivista italiana di Counseling*, Vol. 1.

Piccinino G. (2018) Reflections on physis, happiness, and human motivation. In *Transactional Analysis Journal*, *48*(3): 272–285.

Piccinino G., Natoli Casalegno D. (2010) *Amore limpido* (*Limpid Love*). Trento, Erickson.

Pievani T. (2007) *In difesa di Darwin*. (*In Defense of Darwin*) Milano, Bompiani.

Pievani T. (2011) *La vita inaspettata. Il fascino di un'evoluzione che non ci aveva previsto.* (*Unexpected Life. The Fascination of an Evolution That Did Not Anticipate Us*). Milano, Raffaello Cortina.

Pievani T. (2014) *Evoluti e abbandonati.* (*Evolved and Abandoned*). Torino, Einaudi.

Punset E. (2007) *The Happiness Trip: A Scientific Journey*. White Rivers Junction, VT, Chelsea Green Publishing.

Recalcati M. (2011) *Cosa resta del padre? La paternità nell'epoca iper-moderna* (*What's Left of Father? Fatherhood in the hyper-modern age*). Milano, Raffaello Cortina.

Recalcati M. (2012) *Ritratti del desiderio* (*Portraits of Desire*). Milano: Raffaello Cortina.

Recalcati M. (2013) *Il complesso di Telemaco. Geniori e figli dopo il tramonto del padre* (*The Telemachus complex. Parents and children after the sunset of the father*). Milano, Feltrinelli.

Recalcati M. (2014) *La forza del desiderio* (*The Power of Desire*). Monastero di Bose, Quiqaion.

Riddley M. (2003) *The Red Queen: Sex and the Evolution of Human Nature*. New York, Harper Collins.

Rifkin J. (2010) *The Empathic Civilization*. New York, Jeremy P. Tarcher inc.

Rizzolatti G., Sinigaglia C. (2006) *So quel che fai. Il cervello che agisce e i neuroni specchio* (*I Know What You Do. The Acting Brain and Mirror Neurons*). Milano, Raffaello Cortina.

Rizzolatti G., Vozza L. (2009) *Nella mente degli altri* (*In the Minds of Others*). Bologna, Zanichelli.

Rogers C. (1951) *Client-Centered Therapy. Its Current Practice, Implication and Theory*. Boston, Houghton Mifflin.

Romanini M. T. (1999) *Costruirsi persona* (*Building Yourself Person*). Milano, La vita felice.

Ronson J. (2012) *The Psychopath Test: A Journey Through the Madness Industry*. New York, Riverhead Books.

Ryan R., Deci E. (2017) *Self-Determination Theory: Basic Psychological Needs in Motivation, Development, and Wellness*. New York, Guilford press.

Schellenbaum P. (1990) *The Wound of the Unloved: Releasing the Life Energy*. Dorset, UK, Element Books.

Schiff A., Schiff J. L. (1971) Passivity. In *Transactional Analysis Journal*, 1(1): 71–78.

Schiff J. L. (1975) *Transactional Analysis Treatment of Psychosis. Catextis Reader*. New York, Harper & Row.

Seligman M. (1998) *Learning Optimism*. New York, Pocket Books.

Seligman M. (2003) *Authentic Happiness: Using the New Positive Psychology to Realize Your Potential for Lasting Fulfillment*. London, Nicholas Brealey Publishing.

Sen, A. (2000) *Development as Freedom*. New York, Anchor.

Sennet R. (2012) *Together: The Rituals, Pleasures and Politics of Cooperation*. London, Yale University Press.

Sills C., Hargaden H. (2002) *Transactional Analysis. A Relational Perspective*. London, Routledge.

Skinner B. F. (2011) *About Behaviorism*. New York, Vintage books.

Steiner C. (1966) Scripts and counterscripts. In *Transactional Analysis Bulletin*, 5: 18.

Steiner C. (1971) The stroke economy. In *Transactional Analysis Journal*, 1: 3.

Steiner C. (1974) *Scripts People Live: Transactional Analysis of Life Scripts*. New York, Grove Press.

Stenhouse D. (1974) *The Evolution of Intelligence*. New York, Barnes & Noble Books.

Stern D. (1995) *Motherhood Constellation: A Unified View of Parent-Infant Psychotherapy*. New York. Routledge.

Stewart I., Joines, V. (1996) *TA Today: A New Introduction to Transactional Analysis*. Melton Mombray, UK, Life Space.

Tomasello M. (1999) *The Cultural Origins of Human Cognition*, Cambridge, MA, Harvard University Press.

Tomasello M. (2008) *Origins of Human Communication*. Cambridge, MA, MIT Press.

Tomasello M. (2009) *Why We Cooperate*, Cambridge, MA, MIT Press.

Tomasello M. (2014) *A Natural History of Human Thinking*. Cambridge, MA, Harvard University Press.

Tomasello M. (2019) *Becoming Human: A Theory of Ontogeny*. Cambridge, MA, Harvard University Press.

Ventriglia S. (2011) Il viaggio del copione: storia e sviluppo teorico (The journey of the script: History and theoretical development). In *Neopsiche*, 10: 7–15.

Vercellino Giovannoli C. (2009) *Il gruppo psicoterapeutico (The Terapeutic Group)*. Trauben, Torino.

Watson J. (1930) *Behaviorism* (revised edition). Chicago, University of Chicago Press.

Williamson M. (1992) *A Return to Love: Reflections on the Principles of A Course in Miracles*. New York, Harper Collins.

Winnicott D. W. (1987) *Babies and Their Mothers*. New York, Da Capo Press.

Woollams S., Brown, M. (1978) *Transactional Analysis*. Dexter, MI, Huron Valley Institute Press.

Yalom I. (2002) *The Gift of Therapy: An Open Letter to a New Generation of Therapists and Their Patients*. New York, Harper Collins.

Yalom I. (2017) *Becoming Myself*. Boston, Little Brown Book Group.

Yalom I., Leszcz M. (1970) *The Theory and Practice of Group Psychotherapy*. New York, Basic Books.

Yalom I., Yalom M. (2019) *A Matter of Death and Life*. Redwood City, Stanford University Press.

Zeldin T. (2015) *The Hidden Pleasures of Life: A New Way of Remembering the Past and Imagining the Future*. London, Quercus.

ZoJa L. (2009) *La morte del prossimo (The Death of the Neighbor)*. Torino, Einaudi.

# Index

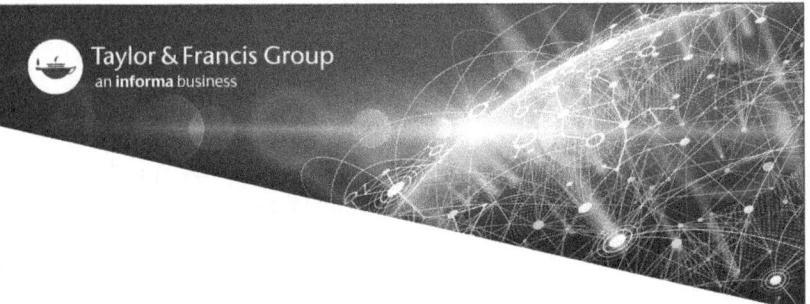
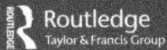
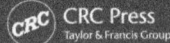